M000299847

Cross of a Different Kind
Cancer & Christian Spirituality

Anthony Maranise, M.A.

With a Feature-Foreword by
Melissa M. Hudson, M.D.

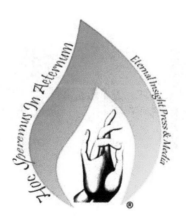

Other Titles by Anthony Maranise:

Sport & the Spiritual Life
The Integration of Playing & Praying

Worth Holding On To

Faith-Filled Fragments

Beyond "I Am"
Meditations on the Gospel of Saint John

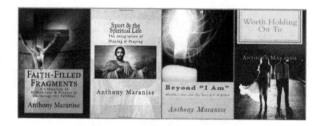

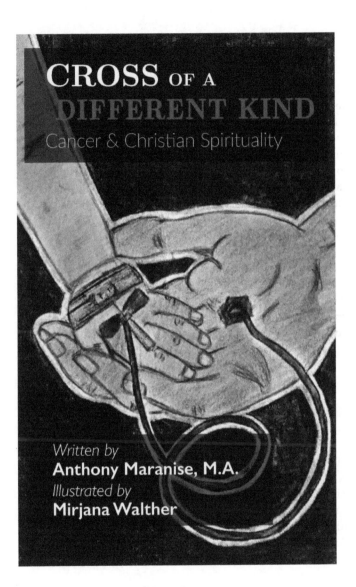

CROSS OF A DIFFERENT KIND
Cancer & Christian Spirituality

Written by
Anthony Maranise, M.A.
Illustrated by
Mirjana Walther

Eternal
Insight
Press

Cover & Interior Illustrations by Mirjana M. Walther

Graphic Design by Breanna Parker

Anthony Maranise can be contacted via email, for academic and/or professional purposes only at amaranis@cbu.edu. Do not add this address to automatic mailing-lists.

Library of Congress Cataloging-in-Publication Data
Name: Maranise, Anthony, author.
Title: Cross of a Different Kind: Cancer & Christian Spirituality / Anthony Maranise
Identifiers: LCCN 2017916616 | ISBN 9780692974148
Subjects: Religion – Christianity. | Spirituality – Christianity. | Health – Diseases & Disorders – Cancer.

Printed in the United States of America

"Your love, insofar as it is from God, is permanent. You can claim the permanence of your love as a gift from God. And you can give that permanent love to others… Those whom you love will not leave your heart even when they depart from you… Those you have deeply loved become part of you."

~ Henri J.M. Nouwen
From *The Inner Voice of Love*

In his <u>Summa Theologica</u>, St. Thomas Aquinas writes, "Music is the exaltation of the mind derived from things eternal, bursting forth in sound."

The persons to whom I have chosen to dedicate this book (see following page) have cemented their places in the eternal depths of my heart, each for different reasons, and all of them positive ones.

That said, there are several lyrical verses which will forever remind me, happily, of them and which, in turn, calls me to thank God for these persons, each time I remember them. What follows are those lyrics:

"…I'll say a prayer so that in my heart you always will be there; This is not goodbye, I know we'll meet again… It's just a 'love you' to take with you until we're home again."
~ Adapted from "This is Not Goodbye" by Sidewalk Prophets

"Say you'll remember me… Say you'll see me again even if it's just in your wildest dreams."
~ "Wildest Dreams" by Taylor Swift

"As the years go flying by, I hope you smile if I ever cross your mind; it was the pleasure of my life and I cherished every time; my whole world, it begins and ends with you."
~ "Highway 20 Ride" by Zac Brown Band

Dedication

To Christ the King, through St. Jude Thaddeus
"Propter vos habito"
Ever my only hope in life's darkest hours

◊

In beloved memory of Sid E. Kraker
July 6, 1992 – November 27, 2016
"Semper meus frater, et Amicus, et Requiescant in pace Christi"
Even your laughter in Heaven gladdens God

◊

In honor of the Illustrator, "Missy" Walther
"Quod in Christi, quid esset bonum et verum, ut semper sit"
With whom I am grateful to have shared in
experience & indelible ink, "the fullness of life"

+

Caritate Dei, Gratias Vobis.

+

On behalf of our charitable beneficiaries, both the author and the illustrator sincerely thank you for your purchase of this true "labor of love."

100% of all royalties and proceeds from the sales of this book will be donated to non-profit charities.

Praise for *Cross of a Different Kind*

"Anthony Maranise's book, Cross of a Different Kind is insightful into the nature of Christian suffering as it finds its meaning in Christ. Suffering for the young, especially cancer victims, always seems so cruel and senseless when there is so much to live for and experience in life. Maranise has captured the essence of suffering as gift when one receives it in Christ and recognizes that one can choose to bear such a burden even in the joy of the moment. Those who suffer have much to teach us about joy in sorrow and its transformative power, if we will but embrace the hope that springs from love. Cross of a Different Kind has something to offer all ages."

- Rt. Rev. Cletus Meagher, OSB
Abbot, St. Bernard Abbey
Cullman, Alabama

"After forty-two days of radiation and now over eleven years in remission, I can honestly say that Maranise's Cross of a Different Kind: Cancer and Christian Spirituality certainly touched my life. Each chapter resonated for me personally. Each chapter reminds me of the different stages that a cancer patient goes through and how faith gives them hope."

- Rev. Anthony F. Rigoli, OMI
Pastor, Our Lady of Guadalupe Church / Shrine of St. Jude
New Orleans, Louisiana

"A 'must read' for anyone who has ever struggled with the griefs and sufferings of this world and asked: 'Why, God?' Anthony Maranise has carried the cross of cancer to find the way of compassion and healing. He shows us what it takes. But he takes us further. Christ's Passion is incomplete without life for all beyond the Cross. In Anthony's ministry, and in the courage and wisdom of those to whom he ministers, we find one faith-filled answer to Christ's call to bring His saving presence to all His sisters and brothers in need."

your life just as did Simon of Cyrene for the Master. As a youngster, Anthony Maranise survived cancer through Our Lord's grace and with the help of the world's leading pediatric cancer center. Now, as a mature Christian, Maranise shares his experiences, strength, and hope in *Cross of a Different Kind* to help readers persevere in their own struggle and to support the lifesaving mission of St. Jude Children's Research Hospital."

- Joe Birch
Lead Anchor
WMC TV, Action News 5 – Memphis, Tenn.

"This book takes every reader to a place that is most meaningful: The very purpose of existence. Maranise does a wonderful job of addressing the universal experiences of persons who encounter cancer, and seamlessly weaves together these difficult topics with the helpful and hopeful insights of Christianity. The book delivers in allowing us to walk the path of our Suffering Savior while simultaneously addressing the struggles the author has endured as a cancer survivor and for all who suffer in general."

- John Acquaviva, Ph.D.
Professor, Wingate University
Author, *Improving Your Body Image through Catholic Teaching & Raising Kids with Healthy Body Image*

"*Cross of a Different Kind: Cancer & Christian Spirituality* offers a deep theological comparison into the suffering endured by Jesus in crucifixion with that of one battling cancer. Maranise demonstrates, through his own painful experience as a cancer survivor, the human suffering Jesus must have endured during His own crucifixion and the physical signs of torture visible even after the Resurrection. The author employs his theological expertise to help readers understand how it is possible for a person to experience pain and suffering and yet still grow in faith and love."

- Didier Aur
Catholic Educator & Jubilee Schools Administrator

"Anthony Maranise's book is the work of a spiritual being on an earthly journey. His cancer diagnosis and survival some 20 years ago set him on a path that has led him closer to God, and empowers him to reach out in hopes of bringing others on their own journeys ever closer to the God of Life. His book touches our hearts, and our lives, as he proclaims God's goodness as experienced through the challenges, sufferings, and yes, even triumphs of the cancer experience. This book is a 'must read' for spiritual renewal."

- Mary C. McDonald, Ph.D.
President, MCD Partners: Education Consultants
Author, *A History with God*

"What initially led me to this book was the title – in that it includes both "Cross" and "Cancer." Belonging to the Community of the Servants of Mary, we believe in standing at the foot of the cross for those suffering in today's world. This book is a <u>must</u> read if you have the privilege of walking the cancer journey with someone. Anthony's personal insights and stories are both touching and invaluable lessons for us all.

- Sr. Linda Hess, OSM
Director, St. Peregrine Cancer & Catastrophic Illnesses Ministry
Omaha, Nebraska

"Cancer made Anthony Maranise vulnerable. In *Cross of a Different Kind: Cancer & Christian Spirituality*, Maranise shares how his vulnerability was transformed by his Christian faith. His honest and thoughtful reflections will assist anyone facing so particular a challenge and it will provide perspective to loved-ones who journey with them. This is a book for all of us."

- Monsignor John Woods
Cathedral Administrator and Vicar for Education
Archdiocese of Canberra and Goulburn, Australia

Table of Contents

Foreword

Cancer, previously considered a uniformly fatal disease, is now curable with more than 60% of adults and 80% of children anticipated to survive at least five years from diagnosis. For some, long-term therapy may be needed to control unresponsive cancer or prevent recurrence. For most, general health typically improves after completion of therapy, however long-term health may be compromised by persistent physical changes, chronic symptoms, and health problems resulting from late-onset toxic effects of therapy. Consequently, cancer patients, even long-term survivors off therapy, may have to accept living with a "new normal" because of physical limitations resulting from cancer or its treatment.

The cancer experience also causes emotional distress to patients and their loved ones as they navigate through the anxiety and uncertainty associated with a potentially life-threatening diagnosis, invasive procedures and toxic treatment, and concerns about relapse and long-term negative health effects of cancer. Persistent cancer-related anxiety and fears have been noted in a significant minority of long-term survivors with negative consequences to their health-related quality of life. Indeed, some cancer patients and their caregivers endorse "re-experiencing" and intrusive memories related to cancer events akin to post-traumatic symptoms. However, emerging research notes minimal distress and disruption in psychological functioning following traumatic events characteristic of resilience. Moreover, the challenges of childhood cancer have been reported to promote psychological growth manifest by enhancement of family and emotional relationships, reprioritization of life goals, and participation in social activism. In my practice, I have been humbled by the growth and resilience of long-term survivors and their families who struggle with and typically overcome the difficulties thrust upon them by cancer. Examples include the family who rallies to support a cognitively impaired brain tumor survivor by keeping him engaged in the family business and community activities. Or the bone tumor survivor who does not let chronic pain and functional limitations following amputation influence his contribution to family and work responsibilities.

What is the path to promoting resilience and psychological growth among individuals experiencing the challenges and uncertainties of cancer? For people of faith, the cancer experience may be accompanied by feelings of anger and abandonment toward God. In others, their faith can facilitate acceptance through identification of newfound meaning in their illness. For all, maintaining a positive outlook and engaging actively in faith-based or spiritual activities provides a path to psychological growth and resilience, irrespective of the individual's outcomes after cancer. In <u>Cross of a Different Kind</u>, Anthony Maranise provides a number of spiritual perspectives, born of his own encounter with childhood cancer as well as his scholastic theological training, as to how faith acknowledges these sentiments and contributes to both emotional and holistic improvement for cancer patients, long-term survivors and their families during periods of hopelessness, helplessness, depression, and anxiety that characterize the cancer experience. I can attest through personal observation that Anthony's reliance on the strength which faith alone provides empowered him to overcome many of the emotionally difficult obstacles of his cancer experience. The insights he shares in <u>Cross of a Different Kind</u> about the role of faith in his personal path to growth and resilience is a must read that will resonate with individuals struggling to maintain inner-strength in the midst of cancer's adversities.

--- Melissa M. Hudson, M.D.
Director, Cancer Survivorship Division
Department of Oncology
St. Jude Children's Research Hospital
Memphis, Tennessee

A Personal Preface from the Author

What follows here below is what you might call "my personal stake" in all of the content that makes up this book. I have encountered cancer personally. I would be remiss did I not mention at the outset that this personal preface of mine is from an article I previously published in a phenomenal publication known as "The Word Among Us." This article was featured in their June 2010 issue.

The year was 1994. I was five years old and on the "little league" soccer team of Holy Rosary Catholic School. I was eager to play, but after only a few moments on the field, my legs would begin to twinge in pain and feel too heavy to run. Alarmed by this and by my persistent cold-like symptoms, my parents took me to the doctor. He found nothing unusual. Three months later, bruises appeared on my legs and thighs, and a blood test revealed that my white blood-cell count was extremely high. I was referred to the world-famous St. Jude Children's Research Hospital in Memphis, Tennessee. Memories from my first visit there are etched in my mind: the smiles of the doctor and nurses who greeted us . . . the seemingly endless tests . . . my equally endless repetition of the only question on my mind that day: "When do we get to go home?". . . the look on my parents' faces when they emerged from their consultation with the specialists. They had just learned that their only child had acute lymphoblastic leukemia, the most common form of childhood cancer.

Being so young, I could tell only that something was wrong. What this would mean in practical terms, though, I began to experience right away. Instantly, I was started on a plan of treatment that would bring me back to St. Jude hospital for intravenous chemotherapy every Tuesday. It would be impossible to count the number of needles used for my blood tests in the two and a half years that followed—the doses of medication I received, the moments of nausea and pain, the prayers offered on my behalf, or the sleepless nights of my parents, family, and friends. But finally, all those prayers to Christ and to St. Jude Thaddeus, "the patron of impossible causes," were answered. On a sunny day in April 1997, I was declared cancer free and have remained so to this day. The arduous fight was over.

All my life, I have been told, "It's something special to be a cancer survivor." But of course, there is an element of mystery in the fact that I survived cancer while so many other people have not. And so, even as I enjoyed living my normal life again, I could not empty my heart of two huge questions: How come God gave me this second chance? What am I supposed to do? I was nearly fourteen when I began to glimpse some answers. It dawned on me that God might be calling me to serve him by serving others as a religious educator. My own faith and love of God had been planted by the teaching I received in my family: from my parents and maternal grandparents, who taught me how to pray, assured me that Jesus was with me in my suffering, and introduced me to saints, including Jude. What a privilege it would be to lead other people closer to God, I thought. And now, some fourteen years later, my hope has been realized. Not only do I have the opportunity to share my faith with others but I can also share my experience with leukemia as a way to encourage them to trust in God.

In all honesty, I don't know if surviving cancer makes me special. But I do know that reflecting on my experience has opened the door to many insights about the Christian life. Some of these thoughts have to do with the virtues of faith, hope, and love, and how they work together.

When we talk about people who have cancer, we often say things like, "He's fighting," or "She's battling it." This always makes me think of how St. Paul urged Timothy to fight the good fight of faith (1 Timothy 6:12). For anyone who has been thrust into combat with cancer—and all the discomfort, pain, and even agony that come along with it—Paul's encouragement takes on special meaning. It's by faith that we believe in Jesus and come to have a personal relationship with him. In the fight against a disease like cancer, this virtue is an anchor in your darkest moments. I remember days when I truly thought that I was going to die. The smiles of family and friends brought comfort, but the only certainty came from faith in Jesus, who said, "I am the resurrection and the life" (John 11:25). Young as I was, this truth spoke to me, and I felt the great peace of Christ that comes along with it. I also experienced the way that faith joins hands with hope, the virtue that "does not disappoint" (Romans 5:5).

Hope strengthens us to place our trust in Jesus' promises and to long for the kingdom of heaven as our ultimate happiness. In this continual looking forward, we trust that God is bringing us closer to this goal and working for our greater good in every circumstance, no matter how bleak things may appear. And so, when cancer's sufferings seem unbearable, something deep within propels you to keep going. You realize that you will reach the end of the pain—either because tomorrow will be better or, in the worst-case scenario, because you know that all earthly sorrows will vanish away once you see Jesus in his glory. This happened to me one day while I was receiving a treatment. Due to an allergic reaction, my breathing slowed down in an alarming way that brought doctors and nurses rushing to my side. I was terrified, but then came a most powerful experience of hope. As I began what I thought would be my final prayers on this earth, I felt a deep trust in God's providence, along with a fervent desire to look into the loving eyes of Christ. That hope sustained me until I was stabilized and the threat was over.

Scripture tells us that "God is love" (1 John 4:8), and Jesus' sacrifice on the cross perfectly exemplifies what that love means: It is to place the interests of others before your own. I am convinced I would have lost my fight against leukemia had it not been for the way my family showed me this kind of love. In every agonizing moment of chemotherapy, as I wrestled with severe nausea or writhing pain, my parents or grandparents were there to soothe me with a cool cloth, a heating pad, and soft words of comfort and encouragement. Continuously, I heard, "We love you" and "We're praying for you," and "What can I do to help you feel better?" My family could have left the bulk of my care to the nurses, but rather than thinking of themselves, they thought of me. What wondrous love! "Your son has seen the face of the Lord," a priest once told my father. I believe he's right. We are all made in the image and likeness of God. Each of us is called to share and grow in the characteristics of Christ the Lord. If "God is love," I have surely seen him through every person who demonstrated Jesus' selfless giving in the way they cared for me. Now it's my turn to show the face of God to others.

Introduction

In 2015, a survey from the United States Center for Disease Control and Prevention (CDC) reported that more than 69% of cancer patients pray for their health (in addition, of course, to medical treatments such as chemotherapy, radiation, and surgical interventions) regularly. While this, in itself, is likely not so surprising, the more startling fact may actually be that this number is *only* 69%. Yet another publication, this time from the American Cancer Society (ACS) in their peer-reviewed academic journal known as <u>Cancer</u>, revealed that cancer patients, as well as survivors who prayed for or about their health generally reported better health later in life. For a person of faith, this is likely not at all surprising given that God, after all, in Judeo-Christian context, and as evidenced in the written recounting of the life, teachings, and works of the incarnate God (Jesus) in the New Testament of the Bible is often shown to be "the Divine Physician," capable of and do accomplishing numerous healings.

It would be morally and ethically irresponsible of me to assure or to promise readers of this short book any sort of cure, better health, or even a miracle as a result of their prayers. After all, I do not know or pretend to know the will of God for all things. I don't think any human person does. He is, after all, far above our human understanding. As a trained theologian, however, I learned both early on and rather quickly that while God's mind is far above and beyond ours, His mind is, nevertheless, like ours. It is only in this way that we can be sure that we have been made *imago Dei*, or "in His own image and likeness." God incarnate in Jesus of Nazareth is a Being of infinite power, knowledge, and love. We, as human beings, are finite – that is – limited in our capacities for power, knowledge, and regrettably, even love. There is quite literally, however, a saving grace in all of this. That brings me to why I have chosen to write this book in my own 20th year of remission from leukemia.

Why I've Written This Book

The answer is simple. I am writing this book because, in one way or another, I have been where you are. Yes, any reader of this book: I have been where you are. I've struggled through cancer and fought for my own life. I've lost dear loved-ones to it; and I have survived it. "Great for you, you braggadocios prig. Rub it in my face," you may think. That is *not* my intention; the furthest thing from it, in fact, as you will soon see for yourself. So, if the tone of this work has thus far "turned you off," perhaps I could politely ask you to give me a chance. Keep on reading.

I've actually got another study for you. In a January 2016 journal article entitled, "The Effect of Prayer on Patient's Health," the authors concluded: "Consistency in the results were found in that prayer, whether petitionary or intercessory, seems to help patients cope more effectively in times of illness and/or crisis." That said, whether you trust in prayer and spirituality's abilities to help you or not – scientific evidence show us that it can and does one way or another. Either the use of prayer and Christian spiritual practices helps one in the prognosis or outcome of their treatment (as discussed in the first study) or it helps in the acceptance of, coping with, and coming-to-terms with one's diagnosis (the results of the second study). Both studies support the inference that prayer and spirituality are conclusively effective in the ways in which they help all persons affected by cancer, whether we understand how this is possible or not.

I wanted to write this book, as one affected in all ways by cancer, as a help to those going through any phase of it: a) having lost loved ones to it, b) those who are fighting through it currently, and c) those who have survived. I lost both of my grandfathers to this "natural evil" (I'll say more on why cancer is labeled as such later); I fought personally through two and a half years of agonizing chemotherapy treatments, procedures, and exams (all of which, though I was a young child when I experienced my confrontation with leukemia, I remember vividly); and last but not least, and only by the grace of God, I've survived. It's been a little over twenty years now since I entered remission and was "counted among the cured," however, nearly every single day since my last chemo treatment, I have feared a relapse or a subsequent diagnosis. Comfort came to me around ten years out when I learned that much of the anxiety I was experiencing and continue to experience is very much directly linked to the traumatic experiences from my youth. A dear friend of mine (and fellow cancer-survivor) and I actually discussed this very thing over lunch one afternoon not too long ago at the time of the writing of this book. Both of us – some years now after our respective treatments – have been diagnosed with anxiety-related disorders of various sorts. For both of us, we experienced symptoms such as fear, worry, loss-of-emotional-stability, etc.; all of which we were able to recognize were far beyond the ordinary concerns and usual worries of life that the general population experiences from time-to-time. While not classified as such, we essentially have a most mild version of PTSD. Though some may think so because of the media's more prevalent reporting, PTSD is *not* something only soldiers who have seen combat can acquire. In fact, elsewhere (see Appendix 1 to this book) I have argued that those in *any* way "touched" by cancer are soldiers in their own ways. But, I digress: while still surely receiving assistance from counselors and other mental healthcare professionals, both my cancer-survivor friend and I have found incredible strength, comfort, healing, compassion, and hope beyond all hope in a relationship with Jesus Christ.

Unashamedly Christian, I trust that God never once left me during my cancer struggles and that He doesn't and never will leave any of us. "Easier said than believed," you might think, but therein is the entire reason I chose to write this book in the first place; namely, because when no one else understood (or even now understands) what I felt, experienced, or prayed… at least for me, Jesus did. And He still does. And He awaits us to only turn to him in confidence and ask for the help we so often desperately need. Faith – more specifically, the <u>practice</u> of that faith, belief, trust, and hope in God incarnate in Jesus Christ (what we call "Christian Spirituality") helped me through my struggle and helps me even now. That said, I hope you will continue to trust and have hope in He who is mercy itself, to help you through your own struggles. As little children often say, and with the most pure of intentions and desires to truly do so, I say now: "I'm just trying to help."

How To Read This Book

The short answer to the question, "How does this book work?" is: "However you want." There's no need to read it from cover-to-cover, unless you want or feel somehow compelled to do so. This book is meant to act as a "field-guide" of sorts for all persons "touched" by cancer and for whom faith also plays a significant role in their lives. I should further explain that phrasing. Throughout the remainder of this book, unless otherwise specifically mentioned in certain circumstances, when I refer to those who are in any way "touched" by cancer, I am referring to all three groups ever affected by it: 1) those who have lost loved-ones to it and who grieve their loss, 2) those who are currently fighting the battle – either personally or who are caregivers, family, or friends of someone fighting it, and 3) those who have survived, but like myself, still realize that life will never be the same – and I would argue, in the best way possible! So, from this brief book, take or read whatever you need.

Though I've been, personally, a member at various points throughout my life of all three groups discussed in this book, I've grown to learn more and more, through both studies and practical chaplaincy experience about the questions, ideas, needs, and concerns – all unique to the experience itself – of all those "touched" by cancer. Let me be clear: those are my qualifications… academia and lived-experience… But, even with those qualifications, I <u>will not</u> be able to answer all of the questions we all have. Allow, then, **_your own_** experiences to supplement what my own contents herein may lack. Make this book your own. But, if you'd humor me, consider this: There is a phrase I was always taught to believe when I first started out as a teacher. It resounds, "If you help only one person in your lifetime of work by what you've done, then you've left the world better than you found it." I hope my book can help you, even if only ever-so-slightly. There is content in each part and chapter, to be sure, but at the end of each of the three parts, there are also "Suggested Spiritual Exercises" and additional resources, inspired loosely by and somewhat akin to those of St. Ignatius of Loyola, but tailored specifically to all cancer-"touched" persons. Always remember this: cancer may very well be an "evil" of sorts, but the Lord – God incarnate in Jesus – experienced, suffered through, and *overwhelmingly conquered* all evil… and because He did, once and for all, in His name and by our identity as believers in Him, so also shall we.

\-   Anthony Maranise, M.A.

March 5, 2017

Our Lady of Blind River Chapel

Gramercy, Louisiana

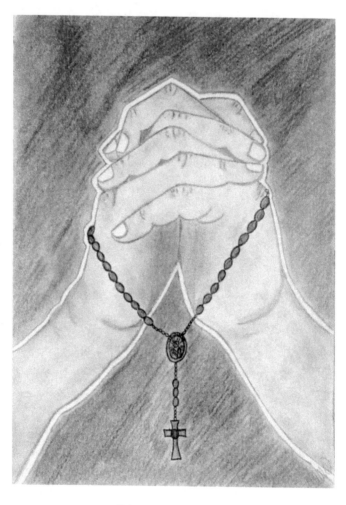

© *Mirjana Walther, 2017*

Part I

For Those Left to Carry On

"Those Who Have Lost Loved-Ones to Cancer"

Chapter 1:
Only the Body, Not the Soul

As I pen this chapter, I feel the weight of sadness from loss. Within the last five months (at the time of this writing), I have lost two people I dearly loved. One, I lost to his passing over from this temporary life to an eternal one; and the other, I lost emotionally. She and I did our best, for over nine months, to work through and maintain our relationship, but alas, a combination of factors not the least of which included simply being in different phases of life made for an unsustainable combination. I say all this because I am so quickly reminded of something a very wise psychology professor and mentor once told me in a lecture of hers. She said, "Our minds cannot tell the difference in sudden losses; whether death or the end of a relationship, we process these things as trauma and our minds and bodies both treat them as grief." I remember this just as clearly as if she was whispering it to me as I type because I took copious notes in her classes. It doesn't truly surprise me at all that I went through both of these heart-wrenching losses as I endeavored to write this book. Though I have experienced loss before (and yes, even some to cancer), God wanted me to feel grief "in the here-and-now" so that I could write to each of you, who may be going through grief yourself, with a heart and mind akin to your own.

What none of us need right now, as well intentioned as those who tell us may be, is to hear another tired cliché. Enough of the "Things will get better," "You'll see them again one day," or "At least they're not suffering anymore" statements! Enough.

People <u>need</u> to grieve and that is perfectly normal, natural, and healthy. How quickly so many are to forget that even Jesus Himself had to grieve. When one of His very best friends, Lazarus, died, Sacred Scripture tells us:

"Jesus wept" (Jn. 11:35).

Weeping, I should note, is not the same as crying. Is it? There is, as so many of us well know, a difference in intensity. We may shed some tears at a sad movie, but to "weep," that is something profoundly deeper and more painful. Whether a death or a break-up, such a response, "weeping," is not only allowed, but it is perhaps one of the most intensely personal and powerful prayers a human being could offer to God. The Psalmist even writes,

"Tears are prayers too. They travel to God when we cannot even speak" (Psalms 56:8).

When, in fact, we cry or cry extremely (this is "weeping"), we are expressing from the innermost depths of our souls the very truth that the person over whom we shed our tears meant a great deal to us personally. We <u>love</u> (note that I don't use the past tense, "loved," here) those persons we have lost and we miss their irreplaceable presence in our lives. Because "God is Love" (1 Jn. 4:8) Himself, Christian theology holds that in any sincere and meaningful expression of love – whether reciprocated or not back to us by the object of our love – there present, is God Himself. As we know, certain losses can be so difficult to process that, as I have both experienced and witnessed in my role as a chaplain over the years, sometimes, we simply cannot find the words to speak into prayer. Some Christians feel guilty about this. If you are one such person, cast off your guilt for this. That is no sin. Your pain is, in and of itself, an unspoken prayer. If you know the grieving who feel this way, encourage them by reminding them that when we cannot even find words to utter in prayer, the incarnate God feels, knows, and accepts the very prayers which silently cry out from the depths of our hurting souls.

Cry it out or even sit in silent stillness, if you must, but be certain that whether in tears or in silence, you are still offering prayers to the God of All Comfort. And even if, at times, we feel as if though He isn't listening, isn't there, or even doesn't care, be further encouraged that He is present, listening, cares, and will turn your sorrow in unspeakable joy. Perhaps some of this sounds like the aforementioned tired clichés that we need to avoid. In that case, allow me to pivot over to the aim, most primary, of this chapter. While the attribution of the following quote to the wise English Christian apologist and famed-writer, C.S. Lewis is sometimes disputed as not having been said by him (as we don't find this in any of his published works), we know not to whom else we might attribute this quote. Nevertheless, it reads:

"You don't have a soul.
You are a soul; you have a body."

The first line there may well shock and surprise some Christians, but let us reflect, even if only momentarily, on its significance – that of the quote as a whole, lest we otherwise take it out of its intended context. In truth, our souls have existed with God longer than we ever have physically existed. God spoke these very Words to the Prophet Jeremiah:

"Before I formed you in the womb, I knew you" (1:5).

If this is true, as our faith proclaims, then somehow, yes, some way, we existed before ever even being of a physical-material-organic-bodily substance. This is the **soul.** We all begin not as the merger of sperm and egg – no – rather, we begin as spirit. We begin with God and to Him we return. The concept of a soul or *the* soul being in any way "ours" is a most distorted view, in the first place. "Our" souls do not now nor do they ever even "belong" to us at all. They belong to their Source and their Origin that is God Himself. We only ever get "our" souls on loan, so to speak. Think of them as a sort of "metaphysical library book." In order to return to their Source, we must care for them, lest we have to "pay a penalty" for the "damages (of sin) incurred" which also may result, if severely enough damaged, in terms of our metaphor, in that which is "on-loan" being unable to return to its Origin. I will trust that these analogies are well-enough understood so that this point need not be further prolonged.

Therefore, since we begin with God as soul, we do not – obviously – cease to be a soul once we receive a body. As the quote states, we "do not <u>have</u> a soul," instead, we "<u>are</u> a soul." Meaning: the most real, most important, most valuable, ever indestructible, indissoluble part of what makes us God's own; what really makes us human has *so little* to do with our physical bodies. Remember: we **are** soul; we only have bodies. In that way, our bodies are merely vessels, fleeting and temporary possessions which ultimately amount to and count for little. So, where, you may wonder, am I going with all of this? I hope to make clear that cancer only affects the body. It does not diminish the soul, which is after all, what we **truly** are. Cancer can take our bodies from us and all the merely mechanical things which cause them to function, but it cannot, does not, and never will be able to make us less real, important, valued, loved, or missed.

Even in romantic fall-outs (so long as their source was in real and authentic love, and not solely based in lust), it isn't the body we miss most, but the memories, the time spent, what we shared, how they understood us better than we can at times understand ourselves and we them, their humor and abilities to comfort, to love, to make and keep promises, their loyalty, their fidelity, and a whole host of other attributes and qualities that are not even traits of the body. We come to love other souls and the saving grace is that souls do not die, do not end, do not hold within them resentment, and above all, return always to God, their Source, to whom our own souls shall return to be forever reunited with those who have "gone before us marked with the sign of faith." They are preparing now the eternal place for our glorious and unending reunion. Oh, how happy will be that day when divided no longer, we are all whole once again in Divine Love.

Chapter 2:
What Kind of "God" Does This?
Pondering the Christological Response

Short answer: One who went through the same thing. But obviously, that doesn't help much just to see in print. There must be more to it, right? Well, there is, but we are going to end up back in the same place – with shades of grey. In yet another quote with disputed attribution, (it is believed that) St. Augustine once wrote:

"God has one Son, but none without suffering."

When I first heard this some years ago, and reflecting on my previous personal losses, I became angry at God. I know! "How dare I!" "How could you!" right? A wise spiritual director once told me that God doesn't mind when we are mad at Him... just so long as we don't curse Him. But, apparently God doesn't mind when we are mad at Him and, in fact, if we are mad at Him, that means we acknowledge His Presence, His Power, and His Supremacy. So, believe it or not, even in our anger, we can pray to God.

Let me put this another way: God actually doesn't mind when we are angry with Him because 1) He gets that we don't understand the fullness of things as He does. Again, we are finite and limited against His infiniteness and limitlessness and 2) He has actually been where we are... and lived to tell about it. From the Cross, God Himself incarnate in His Son, Jesus, screamed out:

"My God! My God, why have you abandoned me?"

For most Christian religious denominations, belief in the Holy Trinity: God the Father, God the Son, and God the Holy Spirit, is a basic tenant of faith and is most succinctly expressed in The Apostle's Creed (or in some traditions, like my own, even more fully in the Nicene Creed). Denominational differences aside, many Christians still run into an existential problem believing that God would: a) subject His only Son to excruciating pain, suffering and death and b) actually descend from Heaven, become His Son (which in its own way, defies all humanly perceptible physical logic), and then, of His own choosing, suffer through such torment. I suppose now is as good a time as any to warn you that I am about to either shock, challenge, bother, or potentially offend you. That said, I must posit these questions:

If God Himself chose, for our sake, to innocently suffer and die, why do we question when it happens to us?

Have we, at some point, come to deserve better than God Himself?

Can we even compare our sufferings to the weight and pain of bearing the sin and suffering of all humanity past, present, and future?

I willingly admit that these are tough, maybe even harsh questions to consider, especially in the midst of one's own personal grief and loss. But, here is my point: As Genesis reports, all human persons are made, fashioned, and created "in the image and likeness of God." If that be so, then shouldn't we almost expect suffering? Once more, there is a saving grace behind all this. In His letter to the Romans, St. Paul, who both saw the Risen Jesus in-person and was converted from unbelief and the persecution of Christians to absolute belief, wrote:

"For if we have been united with Jesus in a death like His, we will certainly be united in a Resurrection like His" (6:5).

God, who Himself, suffered through His Son, also rose – in the flesh and in the Spirit, united to each other in the same Person. If then, we are made "in the image and likeness of God," we are at the same time, made "in the image and likeness" of who God is and once became; that is, His Son, Jesus Christ.

Because of this then, we can come to, even if only ever-so-slightly, answer our own original question: What kind of God does this? That is, allows suffering, cancer's agony, sorrow, and death. What kind of God?

The same One, who, as we so often do, also questioned; dare I say, even "doubted" His very self!

Remember? "My God! My God, why have you abandoned me?" In that moment when, from the Cross in utter humiliation, pain, sorrow, dejection, and shame, God incarnate questioned and doubted Himself. He was even more, in that moment, a part of Himself – more interior to His very self – than His physical pain would have allowed His own knowing. Moreover, the same ancient Christian theologian, St. Augustine once wrote, in his *Confessions*, "You, my God, are more interior to me even than I am to myself." If God is more a part of us than we are to ourselves, then, even should we face pain, suffering, death, heartbreak, despair, or doubt (all things, by the way, known personally to and experienced by God Himself in

Jesus), we can both know, cry out, and intimately relate to the very God who has experienced the same – and even more severe a loss – and know that He does understand where we are, and what we're going through.

Moreover, we know that Jesus' history (and thus God's own because they are One) did and does not end in ultimate death or loss. We are made, for the millionth (and not the last in this book either) time, "in the image and likeness" of the only Being ever to exist that is solely and completely more powerful than death. Because Jesus died, so must we. This is the hard, but unavoidable reality of our human sinfulness. After all, it was our sins that crucified Jesus ultimately (more on that in Chapter 10). However, that death is only temporary and, as we discussed in Chapter 1, only affects the body… for a time. Yes! Even though we must die in body and our soul ever lives on, there will be a day when, just as Jesus Himself did, we, too, will rise from death, overcoming it in a new, glorified body, ever reunited with our soul which never dies.

Jesus died a physical death and rose in a physical body. This is not a metaphor, a spiritual symbolism of any sort, but a reality. Christians believe, as the Apostle's Creed states, "in the Resurrection of the body." That is how God, in Christ Jesus, responds to cancer; to all forms of both natural and moral evil in this life… By sending His only Son to personally experience, endure, and overcome it all. In so doing, God has offered Himself as a self-sacrificial corrective, righting all wrongs of sin, and forever opening to all believers the doors of everlasting life out of which shine the radiance of comfort, mercy, and all that is good.

Chapter 3:
Strength in Support

"We rise by lifting others."
~ Robert Ingersoll

I'm not sure if Mr. Ingersoll (see quote above) is now a Christian or not, but quite frankly, it doesn't matter. The "truth value" of his quote does not diminish based on the frequency with which he tended to defend agnosticism. I bring his quote into our considerations for this chapter because, even if we cannot right now see how it could ever be possible, we can in fact, use our experiences and what we've learned from having lost loved ones to cancer to help others. Now, perhaps I'm rushing things a bit. Maybe you're reading this book in hope of spiritual strength and comfort because you, yourself, have lost a loved-one. In such a case, I cannot emphasize how important it is to seek out (and believe me, you will find) support groups for those of us who have lost loved-ones to such an "evil" illness.

In the Introduction to this book, I mentioned the term, "natural evil" in passing and said I would explain more about what is meant by this term later in the book. That time has come. In the academic-theological appraisal of one of the greatest (if not *the* greatest) impediments to religious faith – that which we call "the problem of evil" – there arises a most perturbing question:

Why would a God of love, who is also all-powerful, allow people He supposedly loves, to suffer?

Theologians have, throughout the centuries of Christian scholarship, come to identify two forms of evil. Again, for emphasis, what generally makes certain things "evil" is that they cause pain and/or suffering (and no, this is not only limited to physicality). Rare exceptions might include side-effects of medications which are used to treat illnesses, certain insect bites, and things of the like... things which reasonable persons might otherwise excuse. The two types of evil which Christian theologians identify, both of which cause suffering of a sort, are what we call:

1) "Moral" Evil and
2) "Natural" Evil.

The differences between these forms of evil, once more according to Christian theology, ultimately comes down to two further-defining characteristics:

a. Causality
b. Morality.

To be certain, "moral" evil is far more sinister as this sort is caused by human persons and is perpetrated against other human persons; the results of which include *any* form of human suffering whether it be physical, emotional, intellectual, or spiritual. Among the examples of various forms of "moral" evil are actions of inflicted by other persons which require of the inflictor, a free-willed choice to cause intentional harm to another person. Some of these choices include: murder, rape, torture, infidelity, lying, deception, the breaking of promises, etc. Because, in one way or another, all of these things are caused by another person and require their choice – willful, even if misinformed as to how – and they result in the suffering, pain, and harm of another person, we can, do, and ought to rightly speak of these actions not simply as "evil," but more specifically so as to emphasize their sinister character as "moral" evil.

On the other hand, the so-called "natural" evils result outside the realm of human or divine cause. So many are quick to blame God when evils occur, particularly "natural" ones because they aren't caused by human hands and, in the thinking of the one who blames, "must come from somewhere." Thus, God often ends up being blamed, labeled, and consequently derided and cursed, for whatever humans are unable to control and for what still causes suffering, sorrow, and pain. But, what about when good occurs and causes pleasure, comfort, and happiness? Are we, then, also so quickly ready to attribute such things to God? A bit of "food-for-thought" in that question. Nevertheless, "natural" evils, instead of being caused by God, have their origin in the original sin of all humanity. Through humanity's own sinful disobedience of God's designs (see the Genesis creation narratives), evil in all its wicked forms, entered the world.

While it is neither the scope nor competency of this book to delve entirely into the whole "problem of evil," let me make this clear: No matter how difficult it is for us to understand on this side of eternity, the God incarnate in Jesus Christ is a pure Being of absolute and perfect knowledge / wisdom, power, and goodness. Furthermore, God, in His infiniteness cannot contradict His very self which is to say more simply, God _cannot, does not,_ and _will never_ cease to be all-knowing, all-powerful, and all-loving. That said, as difficult to swallow as it may be, we must concede that evil, particularly the more inexplicable of the two types –

"natural" – exists in this world, **_not_** as punishment from God for human sinfulness, but rather as a result of a world originally created in perfection, but corrupted by human sin. While Jesus' sacrifice has once and for all corrected the eternal impact of such corruption, the world will not be made perfect once more until Christ the King, in glory, returns and ushers in "the new Heaven and the new earth" (see several mentions throughout the Biblical book of Revelation). Perhaps, as I assume for one suffering through a loved-one's loss, that answer seems inadequate, or even arouses further anger or confusion towards God. In such a case, where our human knowledge leaves us confounded in comprehending the things of God, I've always found the solution given by the philosopher and mathematician, Blaise Pascal, to be of help. He argued (and mind you, I am paraphrasing here) that he'd rather live life believing in God (and all that means) only to arrive at his death to discover no God rather than to live his life believing that there is no God only to arrive at his death and discover that God is and always has been, and as a result, have to face the judgment of One whose existence he would long have denied.

We have, to this point, discussed what makes certain evils either "natural," that is, they are not caused by human or divine means, but still pain and suffering occur. "Natural" evils, for example, include: tornadoes, aneurysms, earthquakes, and things of the like… and, lest we forget, for our purposes, cancer. Previously, I mentioned that God does not give us, our loved ones or anyone cancer (nor is He the cause of any "natural," and certainly not any "moral" evil). However, there does seem to be – surely I am not the only one to have observed this – something about cancer that makes it tougher to "accept" and to cope with than, say, a random terrorist attack. For this answer, we must revert to considerations of morality. In "moral" evils, we always reflect (typically after their having already occurred) on ways in which there could have been human intervention to have stopped or prevented the action itself. It is the inexplicable randomness of "natural" evils that becomes so difficult for us to process through. If we cannot "blame" a particular human person, a general "gut-reaction" is to blame God. As human beings, we feel ever-compelled to assign responsibility and culpability to negative acts. This is one of our more unfortunate coping-mechanisms. Take this as an example: Several persons smoke their entire lives; multiple packs per day. But, out of that group, only one contracts terminal lung cancer. This, conceivably, is not of the moral culpability of the smoker, since as an action in and of itself, the act is amoral. Generally, no other person forces the individual to smoke and as we have previously discussed, God is not the cause of evil because it would contradict His own nature. Therefore, how must we explain why one person, engaged in a similar lifestyle as a group of others, would contract and perish from such an illness? When you discover the answer to that one, please send me a note.

Our discussions of "moral" and "natural" evil have set the stage for two critical points which, apart from the (at times) long-winded explanations, will, at last, tie this chapter back to its original intent. If you will recall (and it may well require some looking-back), earlier in this chapter, I emphasized the importance of locating and seeking to participate in a cancer-affected persons' support group. Cancer, as a "natural" evil is **unpredictable**, **unexpected**, and generally, affects all its victims in vastly **different** ways. Because of this, many cancer-affected persons (including the loved-ones left to carry on who have lost someone they dearly cared for to the illness) crave stability and "sameness." Within support groups, there exist other persons just as frightened, confused, and longing for stability as you are. The uniqueness of the cancer-experience ***demands*** not merely the attempts of persons who want to understand what you are going through, but who do so by having lived a similar sort of experience. For this reason, we ought to endeavor to seek out not simply any ordinary grief support group, but one which specifically deals with cancer-related losses. Certainly, any support is better than none at all, especially when first learning to cope with the loss, and so we shouldn't shy away from group support if we are only able to find a general grief support group. I merely make the distinction because, as others who have experienced cancer face-to-face will themselves report: "It is an illness unlike any other." Facing the "behemoth-of-loss" as a result of cancer challenges each person differently – to be sure – but, healing and hope can and even often do come from the supportive efforts of others who have been through similar circumstances.

While there are so many different types of cancer, all the forms have a unity not only in pathology (that they are all known to medical professionals to involve abnormal cell growth with potential to invade and spread to other areas of the body), but also, as previously noted, in their abilities to cause suffering, in their unpredictability and in their unexpectedness. That human beings can and do experience these "natural" evils certainly presents occasions wherein faith will be tested, but the old maxim ever rings true:

There is strength in numbers.

Do not be afraid to seek God in the comfort of others who have been where you are. If no grief support groups exist where you are or perhaps more specifically, no cancer-loss grief support groups, perhaps God, the Divine Physician is calling you to begin one so that He, through you, can heal hurting hearts.

Chapter 4:
"We Believe in the Resurrection"

Our fourth chapter takes its name from a line in The Apostle's Creed. This is the general statement of beliefs upon which all Christian religious denominations agree. Toward the end of this statement of beliefs, which is in itself, also a prayer, is written the phrase that lends itself as the title for our chapter. In full, it reads:

"I believe in the resurrection of the body and in life everlasting."

As Christian persons, especially we who have experienced loss of loved-ones – whether to death or emotional separation – this statement and likely several other phrases from The Creed are so much more than mere words or even comforting reassurance. Certainly, they are these things, but for us, they are also hope based on and in the unfailing Word of God Himself.

Before proceeding further, there are a few things I'd like to make clear at the outset. Many Christians have a fundamentally distorted and inaccurate understanding of the very beliefs we profess in The Apostle's Creed. In order for this chapter to have a meaningful impact on the grieving, the hurting, and the suffering, it is **crucial** that we understand what we believe, particularly as it relates to Jesus' Resurrection… and moreover, what it means for us and for our loved-ones. First and foremost, we must acknowledge that Jesus' own Resurrection from the dead not only occurred, but that it occurred on this earth and that it occurred in the physical medium of a human body like our own. True, Jesus was given a new, glorified body at His Resurrection (and this accounts for the reasons why He wasn't immediately recognizable to persons like Mary Magdalene or the persons on the road to Emmaus; see Jn. 20:1-16 and Luke 24:13-35, respectively), but even this new and glorified body contained "the wounds of salvation" (remember: "Doubting Thomas" even put his fingers into the nail marks). This tells us, simultaneously, not only about Jesus, but about ourselves. Yes, us! St. Paul even tells, "For if we are united into a death like Jesus' (and by this he means a physical, bodily death), then we shall certainly also be united in a Resurrection like His (and by this, St. Paul means a physical, bodily rising again – nevermore to face physical death again **_and_** we get a glorified body **_and_** we get to walk this earth again in that glorified body before the end of the world) (cf. Romans 6:5, with my explanations).

Now, maybe that seems outrageous to you or a belief and Truth you've never before been exposed to, heard, or accepted, but good St. Paul has even more to say. He reminds us of how pivotal Jesus' Resurrection (and what it promises and means for us) truly is when, to the Corinthians, and to all of us, he said:

"If Christ has not risen, then our message is invalid and even our faith is useless" (15:14).

Those are pretty strong words from the Apostle, but they are truly significant. See, if Jesus would have simply died and stayed dead, then that also would have meant that everything He taught, said, and promised would have also died the death of a liar. But, certain in faith (and here might I recommend to you for reading and prayerful reflection, a beautiful and very short book by Lee Strobel entitled, *The Case for Easter*) and even in evidence (see Strobel's investigatory book), Christ **IS** truly risen as He promised. Moreover, because He rose, so also shall all of us – and our loved ones – who have come to believe in Him. The Catechism of the Catholic Church has this to say of bodily resurrection:

"By death, the soul is separated (temporarily) from the body, but in the resurrection, God will give incorruptible life to our body, transformed by reunion with our soul. Just as Christ is risen and lives forever, so shall we all at the last day" (§1016).

Whether Catholic or not, such a description of the salvific work of Jesus' death and Resurrection, with particular importance on its impact for us and our loved ones, ought to instill even the faintest glimmer of hope. But still even, there is more. Many of us become so deeply saddened by our losses – whether by death, emotion, or otherwise – because we fear never seeing our loved ones again. Because the impact of loss is often so severe on us, Jesus, in all Divine foresight speaks of something for us to both ponder and look forward to. He said,

"So now you feel anguish and are sorrowful, but I will see you again and your sorrow and grief will be turned into joy; and no one will take your joy from you" (Jn. 16:22).

Jesus promised His Apostles and all of us that we will see Him again. If our loved ones are with Jesus, we have reason to be sure that in seeing Jesus where He is, we will also see and be forever reunited with our lost loved-ones in the resurrection. Christian theology (scripturally expressed in Revelation) teaches of "a new Heaven and a new earth" because, in the work of the Holy Trinity, God will "make all things new" (21:5). Read that once more. "***All things***," says the God of all that is! Our bodies, our loving relationships, our hearts once broken, whatever an form of evil has taken from us... all these things will be made new; that is, <u>not</u> simply restored, once again made whole, reconciled, or resolved – no. Instead, all of those things in perfection, for all eternity, and no longer being subject to loss, sorrow, pain, or shame. This is the faith we profess!

In our darkest moments, when our losses seem nearly unbearable, we must interiorly summon the strength (even if angry at God – which He understands, by the way, or doubtful of His goodness – which He also understands) not to be consumed in despair such that we lose faith completely. Because, then, in so doing, we may also grow apart from those we have already lost, but who are with God in the results-fulfilled of their own faith. They await our arrival and the great reunion, but only when our earthly work is finished. Until then, we press-on in hope, proclaiming those words which **quite literally**, to us at least, mean everything:

"We believe in the resurrection of the body and in life everlasting. Amen."

Chapter 5:
Continual Communication

Allow me, if you will, to open this chapter with a very blunt, but no less true statement: Anyone who advises, cautions, or tells you not to continue communicating with your lost loved-ones fundamentally misunderstands Christianity! Of course, there is importance in developing and utilizing the proper means to an end, in this case. As Christian persons, we should most certainly **avoid** all "dabbling" in séances, psychic mediums, the use of Ouija-boards, and things of the like to attempt to "communicate" with those who have "gone before us marked with the sign of faith." However, there is no wrong, sin, or immorality in continuing to talk to our lost loved-ones through prayers directed to God. Our loved-ones – the dead, who now reside where God does or our lost, but still living loved-ones, who still bear Christ's Spirit as do we – must never be thought of as "gone for good." As we touched on in Chapter 1 of this work, all human persons are so much more than physical beings. Above all, we are spiritual and are endowed with a soul. Souls don't cease interaction merely because the embodied vessel in which we came to know them is no longer a usual fixture in our lives. Souls still know us, love us, and love to hear from us – and always with God's permission – even intervene and intercede for us.

Tainted no longer by sin, sorrow, or the limits imposed by such, souls, having seen and personally experienced the unfathomable depths of God's merciful love and tender compassion, now only see in us the best we have to offer. Souls see us now only, as my wise theological mentor used to say, "Through grace-healed eyes." When we are deeply missing our loved-ones, they know quite well. When we "sense" their benevolent presence with us, this is not by accident. Why, then, shouldn't we communicate prayerfully – always – with those we came to know and love in this life? The great and ever-optimistic Doctor of the Church, St. Francis de Sales, is known to have written about the depths of love's effect on our human lives and its transcendent ability to endure even beyond the "shadows of death." In his remarkable spiritual classic, "Introduction to the Devout Life," De Sales writes:

*"They (*our loving relationships*) begin here which is sure to endure forever there (*or in Heaven*)."*

This being so, as we should trust it to be, we can and ought to continue, even after loss, speaking to our beloved ones in prayer to God. That there is a rich and very deep history of veneration and intercession of the saints is evidence, further, as to the importance and validity of such a spiritual practice.

Human souls, when separated from the body at death, do not in fact (as cartoons may have misled us), become angels. In fact, we, having had to endure the trials of earthly life, actually upon passing from this world and entering Heaven, become saints; that is, even higher than the angels. Various Church Fathers from Augustine to Tertullian have endorsed this understanding, however, this work has not the space or time to treat all such references. I mention all of this to remind you, most especially, of what cancer cannot, does not, and never will be able to take from any of us; and that is the soul. Since the souls of all (living and dead) are "on loan" from God, we can find some consolation, certain in the knowledge that God understands our need to speak to and continue to communicate with those we have come to know and to love in this life. Did not Jesus Himself shout into the tomb of His own friend, Lazarus? So, to whom or what was Jesus speaking when He said, "Lazarus, come out!" Was it to a lifeless corpse or to the ever-present soul of His human, yet departed, friend? The answer, in case there was any question, is the latter.

Now, I, of course, don't say all of this to in any way assert that we can call the dead back to life. After all, we aren't God. However, what we can glean from this is that just as Jesus Himself called out to His own dear friend's soul, so also, through Jesus, and in His name, we can call out in prayer to the souls of our own lost loved-ones. We can… and I would advise, for the sake of our own mental and spiritual sanity… we should. Leaving things unsaid – emotions "trapped up" within us – is a path towards self-destruction. We must "let out" our sorrows, our hopes, our longings, and our joys to those we love. Pray. Cry. Call-out to them, but don't call them back from where they are. They are at-peace now, before God, and free from all sorrow. Yes, we love and miss them, but perhaps C.S. Lewis, in his _A Grief Observed_, said it best:

"How wicked it would be, if we could, to call the dead back… 'I am at peace with God.'"

After all, isn't it that very peace and happiness we want for those we love most of all?

Suggested Spiritual Exercises & Further Resources
Part I

1) Assess your soul.
>*- Are you at peace with your loss?*
>*- If so, go visit them at their resting place.*
>*- If not, write them a letter. Go grab some helium-filled balloons and attach your letter to them. Send it skyward with a prayer.*

2) Read the "Passion Narratives" in the Gospels.
>*- The "Passion Narratives" are the accounts of Jesus' own suffering and death.*
>*- Gaze upon an image of Christ crucified and know that just as we suffer, so did God Himself. Know further that He overcame it and so shall we.*

3) Find and join a support group for those who have lost loved-ones to cancer.
>*- If one doesn't exist in your area, do you think maybe God is calling you to be its founder for your benefit and others?*

4) Read Lee Strobel's *The Case for Easter* **OR** pray The Apostle's Creed.
>*- If you choose the second option, when you get to the part of the prayer which states, "I believe in the resurrection," add in your loved-one's own name there.*
>*- For example, "I believe in the resurrection of Joyce's body," and continue with the prayer to the Amen.*

5) Talk, in prayer to God, about your loved-ones.
>*- Talk to them personally even, but in Jesus' name. Ask*

them to help you through your grief and sadness.

6) Visit mygriefangels.org to search for cancer-loss support groups near you.

7) Consider reading *A Grief Observed* by C.S. Lewis.

8) Consider engaging in art-therapy. Search for and contact your local mental health providers for more.

9) Visit cancer.net; from their drop-down menu, click and explore the "Coping with Cancer" tab.

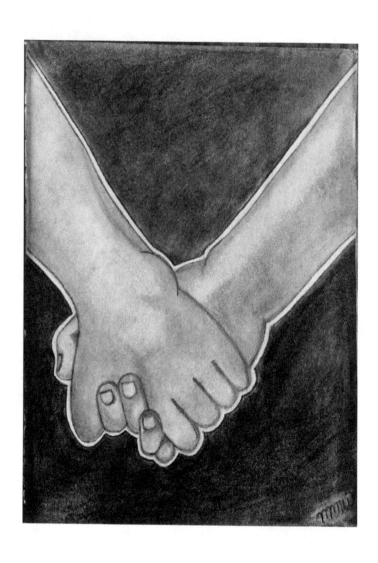

© Mirjana Walther, 2017

Part II

Fighting the Good Fight

"Those Who Are Currently Battling Cancer"

Chapter 6:
The Language of Combat

When doing my background research for this book, I read quite a thought-provoking piece in *The Guardian* entitled, "Cancer is Not a Fight or Battle." In the editorial, the writer, who had an unnamed terminal cancer herself, took issue with the terminology often used to describe someone's dealing with their diagnosis. Going so far in her opening line as to say,

"She lost her brave fight. If anyone mutters these words after my death, wherever I am, I will curse them."

Admittedly, as both a cancer survivor and as one who has both lived the experience of cancer pain and treatment and lost loved-ones to it, I can say that I was at once "off-put" by that writer's statements, and to some degree, I remain to be, but then I thought, "Isn't that what good writing does; namely, challenges us?" So, I read on.

It was ultimately the "language of combat" she took greatest issue with. Her insistence was not at all illogical, to be sure. I even began to understand her point-of-view in some instances, though I must respectfully disagree with her general conclusions. In one of her most poignant arguments, the writer expresses how she doesn't wish to be remembered as a "loser" or as a "failure" should she pass away from her cancer; hence her aversion to the use of the phrase, "She lost her brave fight" (as mentioned above). Nobody likes to lose; much less do we like to lose loved-ones. Those of us currently dealing with a cancer diagnosis certainly don't want to lose. That such language might provoke a similar thought process in others as it had within her was the author's primary point of concern. While her editorial article raises several valid others, for our purposes, we will only be taking up two; the first having already been mentioned.

In her second most compelling argument, she speaks of bravery in the face of cancer. The author writes,

> *"Bravery implies a choice... I didn't choose to be affected by cancer."*

I feel it's safe to say that none of us choose it. From this statement, she goes on to criticize what constitutes authentic bravery as opposed to the perception thereof. While I understand the unique perspectives of her arguments, I cannot gloss over the Truth; and for we who are Christians, we believe as Karl Barth once wrote,

> *"Truth is a person."*

That Person is, of course, the same One from whose lips ever emanate those words,

> *"I am the Way, the Truth, and the Life"* (Jn 14:6).

So, whereas the author of the editorial piece we have been discussing offered one perspective or "way," let us consider not only "another way," but **The Way** to understand the "language of combat" used for cancer.

Recall her first objection to the language of "loss," "defeat," "victory," "failure," or even "fight." St. Paul, on numerous occasions in his letters, uses similar phrasing, and almost always is his use of such language meant as metaphor for a greater and certainly abstract, but no less real purpose. One of St. Paul's most well-known of these metaphors is an encouragement to Timothy wherein he writes:

"Fight the good fight of faith" (1 Tim. 6:12).

Paul is not, here, encouraging Timothy to physically assault persons into believing in Christ, but instead uses this metaphorical phrase to emphasize that perseverance and endurance in faith – much like the trials of cancer – is not easy and will often times require struggle, as would a physical altercation ("a fight"). Sure, this isn't the cheeriest of thoughts, but it is reality nonetheless. Better we know at the outset so as to, even if at least in some way, ready ourselves for what must be endured.

Even before Paul, we hear use of the "language of combat" as metaphor. Jesus Himself directly tells us:

"In this world, you will have troubles, but take courage, for I have overcome this world" (Jn. 16:33).

Jesus not only speaks of this trouble and this victory (read: "overcome"), but He actually goes a step further and shows us. He leads by example. Because of the complexities of a cancer diagnosis, in that it has a way of affecting us on a multidimensional level, it is simply easier to utilize metaphorical language when referring to it. But, once again, I emphasize: merely because we use language which is metaphorical, this does not trivialize the severity or even complexity of the concepts to which we refer. Cancer, of any sort, is difficult; therefore, we must prepare for a "fight" or a "battle." It will cause us "trouble," to be sure, but with the help that comes from the light of faith, the care of our medical professionals, and the support systems we either have (family, friends, etc.) or seek out (support groups, mental health professionals, or faith-leaders), we can and will "overcome."

The author's second primary objection, you may recall, had to do with the concept of bravery. However, it is this skewed perception of bravery that the Truth in the Person of Jesus corrects. She mentioned not having been brave because "bravery implies choice" and she didn't choose to get / have cancer. Once again, no one chooses that willingly, but bravery consists in the choice to respond (and how one goes about doing so) to the cancer diagnosis. We all, when diagnosed, could say to ourselves, "No, I refuse treatment and so I know what my fate will be." And while I actually do know persons who have chosen this option – which is in its own way, brave beyond my own personal comprehension, I contend that perhaps an even greater display of bravery is when one chooses the option to voluntarily subject oneself to treatment (especially if experimental) as in so doing, there is a great deal of uncertainty. Will this work or won't it? Fear of the unknown is one of the greatest causes of clinically-diagnoses anxiety-disorders throughout the world. Cancer patients, either in refusing therapy (which I do not suggest), or in choosing it voluntarily are faced ***daily*** with that very fear of what is unknown.

Even still, there is another dimension: What of those who enter research-based or experimental treatment protocols? The fact that cancer patients rarely, if ever, expect such a truly "evil" diagnosis is also further evidence of their bravery. Even soldiers and military service personnel are trained in what to potentially expect in battle. We, who endure or have endured cancer diagnoses, never saw it coming. No preparation. No training. Yet, one way or another, we persevere. And _that_, dear friends, is always a choice. Did Jesus, in whose image we are all made, necessarily have to choose the cross? Of course not. He is God. However, He freely chose to embrace and submit to the agony of the cross for our sake. Surely, if we cannot count as brave One who freely chose such suffering... to whom can we? Furthermore, I believe there is something to be said about the author's (of the editorial article earlier in this chapter) perception of reality in terms of how she views potentially being remembered as a "loser," or as one "defeated" by her cancer.

Once more, for a uniquely Christian spiritual assessment of her view of being remembered as "defeated" or as "losers" in our "battle, should she or any of us ever succumb to cancer, we turn to the wisdom of St. Paul. In his letter to the Philippians, he writes these words:

"To live is Christ, and to die is gain" (1:21).

In my years of theological training, I have learned on a number of occasions that knowing something and actually believing it are two entirely different, yet, not unconnected things. Paul's phrase, at face-value, may seem perplexing to know or understand. The Christian philosopher and mathematician (whom we spoke of earlier in this book), Blaise Pascal, often suggested that there are merely some things which the mind alone cannot ever know, but which can only come to be understood in and by the heart; that is, as illuminated by faith. Belief, then, becomes the necessary prerequisite for understanding. Paul's phrase is like this. "To live is Christ" means that we have life at all only through "the

Life" Himself, and out of love for the One who at once laid down His own life for us, giving us life in the process, we ought to live in a way which imitates His examples and is devoted to His service.

In this human life, with its joys and comforts; its sorrows and pains, we can still see, feel, experience, and talk to God who lives and loves through His human creation who are bearers of His image. Also at our disposal, to give us strength to "fight the battle" for our lives, we have Christ's Word as well as prayer and the Sacraments. The latter portion of Paul's aforementioned statement reads, "and to die is gain." One day, hopefully ushered into the fullness of His Presence after having "done our best" in this life, we will stand face-to-face and experience the penetrating gaze of Divine Love as we lock eyes with Love Himself. See, then, what we gain? The fullness of eternal Presence, Life, and Communion with Jesus answers all lingering or confusing questions we may ever have experienced in this earth-bound life; it is perpetual relief from all pain, reunion and reconciliation with all those we have loved or lost. It is a glorified body free from decay or distress; and our own share in the resurrection. So, with all respect to the author whose piece we have discussed throughout this chapter, succumbing to cancer would never make us "defeated," or a "loser." Quite the contrary actually, in that "we are more than conquerors through Him who loves us" (Romans 8:37).

Chapter 7:
Dealing with Diagnosis

I was only five years old when I was diagnosed with acute lymphoblastic leukemia (ALL). I often receive skeptical glances from people when I tell them that, even from such an early age, "I can remember that day and its events in vivid detail." One simply doesn't forget, no matter how many years pass, when something utterly life-changing occurs. You, too, will never forget your own date-of-diagnosis (or that of your loved ones). But, I can promise that over time, you will come to accept that memory as part of you, even if like myself, you recall portions of it daily. For me, and I imagine for you as well, one of the most difficult facets of cancer diagnosis is the immediacy within which nearly every aspect of your life as you previously knew it changes. Certain changes are welcome; this we know, and usually those are the ones we invite ourselves, or at least ones for which we are able to prepare.

Cancer is never a willing or a welcome choice; and it is certainly not a welcome change. Though changes in the ways to which we have become accustomed to living are inevitable, I would be remiss were I to neglect to remind you of the things cancer cannot change. Certainly, the diagnosis, pains, and circumstances may shake your faith, even if only temporarily, but cancer does not change who God is – that is, a Being of absolute love, care, concern, and compassion. Cancer does not change your innate value as a human person fashioned in God's own image. It cannot limit your capacities to love or even to hope nor can it rob you of your soul. It cannot stifle your imagination, your creativity, or your dreams… and yes, while it may change you in a number of ways, you retain the abilities to choose how, in each and every moment of your struggle, you will respond to the adversities which come your way.

The aim of this chapter is to generally prepare you to wrestle with three of the most frequently encountered spiritual and existential questions and struggles that cancer-patients tend to encounter along the way. Let me be clear that the three we will be discussing in this chapter by no means comprise the whole of what would otherwise be an exhaustive list. Moreover, if I do not address the questions or concerns most pertinent to you or your loved one (either in this chapter or throughout various phases in the rest of the book), then attribute to me that lack, and please know that it is okay (even encouraged) that you seek both spiritual and emotional assistance beyond what I offer within these pages. Theologian and cancer-experienced though I may be, there is no one, save for the Lord, who has every answer. However, He does call each of us to touch hearts and we cannot possibly accomplish such an undertaking without the help and inspiration of the Holy Spirit. We are all "called" to different means of helping others using gifts that come from the same Holy Spirit, so, as you go forth in dealing with your (or your loved-one's) cancer diagnosis, certainly, use this book as it helps you, but by all means, reach out to others to help you in what may be absent in this work.

That said, let's consider, through the lens of Christian spirituality, those three most frequently encountered spiritual and existential questions faced by those with cancer. Oh yes, one more thing before we get to those: I selected these three for inclusion as I found these to be continuously recurring themes in the course of more than three years of practical experience working to assist in the spiritual care of cancer patients in an inpatient, hospital setting.

1) *"I'm having a tough time praying right now because I feel so upset with God for giving me / my loved-one cancer. Is God going to punish me even more or be mad at me for being mad at Him?"*

To which, I would reply:

"First of all, many cancer patients, it is true, believe that God is punishing them in some way through their illness. God does not "give you cancer." This is <u>not</u> the God in Jesus Christ that we know and love and serve. Christian theology teaches and speaks, in fact, of "the God of all Comfort" (2 Corinthians 1:3-4). Through our earthly pains and adversities, we must cling to this comforting and consoling God. Despite what you may recall or be inclined to argue based in the Old Testament details of God, the importance of context is worth recollection here.

In the Old Testament, no one had ever seen God in the flesh and so coming to personally know and/or relate to Him was accomplished through interior locutions, visions, or the words of prophets. The only way for human creation to come to know the sorts of behaviors God valued was for Him to "correct" human waywardness by means of punishment. However, when God, in the splendor of the Incarnation, became human in Jesus, the world no longer had to relate to God in the abstract, but could come to do so, at long last, "in the flesh." The incarnation, Jesus' obedient life, His Passion, sacrificial death, and Resurrection never "replaced" the Old Testament way of being or His expectations of relating to Him. However, "the Christ event" (that is, the aforementioned series of events in the life of Jesus Christ) fulfilled the previous expectations of the Old Testament and exceeded them all. No longer did persons need punishment to know the sorts of things God values or detests. In the fullness of God incarnate in

Jesus, humanity has a tangible example of how to behave, act, and most importantly, love.

That said, God does not punish – not on this side of eternity – or in the one to come. He is Love itself (cf. 1 Jn. 4:8). Moreover, because God became human in Jesus, there is no human emotion He misunderstands or misconstrues. It is perfectly fine to be "mad" or "upset" at God in your misunderstandings or in your sufferings. He "gets it." The important thing is not to remain in that anger towards Him and to, after some time, persevere in prayer, even when it is difficult. He won't "further punish" you because He is not punishing you in the first place. Moreover, He will not be "mad" at you for being (hopefully only temporarily) "mad" at Him. Whether you understand now or later, you actually aren't "mad" at God because He didn't "do this" to you (see Ch. 3) and He knows that. Return to communicating with Him in prayer when you are ready. He waits with open arms."

2) *"This cancer treatment is going to make (or has made) me bald and/or lose (or gain) a lot of weight; lose a limb or incapacitate me in some way. Who will ever again love me romantically when I am this way?"*

To which, I would reply:

"Have you so quickly forgotten in Whose image you are made? True enough, though, is your concern. Everyone wants to feel, in today's world, "sexy," or "pretty," or "attractive" in and of themselves as well as for others, but what, in this way, we have begun to do, is forget how very little image really matters. When this life is over, we won't be taking our physical beauty, "sexiness," or "attractiveness" into Eternal Easter. In fact, all we will be taking with us is the extent to which we have had faith, held to hope, and loved. The ways in which and to whom we exercised those virtues follows us eternally.

Do we no longer strive after what endures forever? Have we become so consumed by desire for instant gratification that we would so be willing to risk the temporary for the eternal? If any of these answers are "yes," then perhaps our concern isn't so much whether or not others will "love" us, but instead more a matter of whether or not we love ourselves as we should. Genuine love has nothing to do with finding others attractive or even feeling "in-love" with them. Christian theology, everywhere demonstrates this reality, and shows us that love is only authentic insofar as it requires an intentional choice. Now, to be sure, I am certainly "one to talk." Believe me; every break-up I've ever endured (whether of my own choosing, a mutual agreement, or not), I always interiorly questioned whether or not some "aspect beyond my control" (read: "what cancer did to me") had something to do with why it didn't work out. And even if it did (whether my heightened anxiety, my physical appearance, or otherwise), the sin of judgment then rests not with us, but on whomever makes about us such a superficial decision.

As cancer patients, we offer to others, whether they realize it or not, a perspective through which "the world" can seldom clearly see. We learn to see others in the very positive light in which we also hope and crave to be seen by them… a way similar to that in which God sees us… as having been "fearfully and wonderfully made" (Psalms 139:14)."

3) *"I actually feel like I'm handling all of this cancer stuff much better than my family. In fact, I feel like my illness and the extra care I require is driving them further apart. What do I do?"*

To which, I would reply:

"Believe it or not, a fairly decent percentage of cancer-patients when initially diagnosed or in their early treatment stages take up a rather entitled "I deserved to be selfish for a bit" sort of attitude. Both psychology and spiritual direction are in agreement

that such a response is actually perfectly normal as one comes to cope with the "newness" and understandably relatable "outrage" that accompanies such tragic news. However, over time, to really begin to emotionally and spiritually heal, we would do well, in the imitation of Christ, to divert our attention, even in the midst of cancer-struggle, towards others and away from ourselves.

There is a therapeutic-maxim in both positive psychology and pastoral counseling as well as spiritual direction which goes, "Helping others helps us." For the cancer patients so concerned in the midst of their own struggles and sufferings about people _not_ themselves, it is clear that they have already begun to heal... at least emotionally, spiritually, and existentially. Many are misinformed that "grief" is something only experienced by those who have experienced the passing of a loved-one in death. Not so. Grief, in its own ways unique to each person, is experienced in any phase or period of loss or adjustment in life. We can and must "grieve" the loss of or changes to whatever brought us happiness. When persons emotionally separate, one or both parties "grieve" the lost relationship; when a child experiences the divorce of parents, the child "grieves" a change in the familial dynamic; and when we are diagnosed with cancer, though we are very much alive and "fighting," we still must "grieve" the necessary changes to the lives we have been used to prior to our diagnosis. Perhaps we "grieve" how tired we get now so easily or the hair that "chemo claimed" from us.

Traditionally, it has been taught that there are five stages of grief: denial, anger, bargaining, depression, and acceptance. We have learned that grief is not nearly as organized and linear as to follow these "phases" in order. In fact, sometimes, multiple "phases" as there indicated can be experienced together, or some can be entirely skipped. When, as cancer patients, we feel that initial draw immediately after diagnosis to be self-centered, we are responding in grief via a hybrid of both denial and anger. However, when we reach the point wherein we have become more concerned about others (such as how our family is handling our *own diagnosis), it is ultimately safe to say that we have moved beyond self-centeredness (and anger) and into selflessness (and thus closer to total acceptance).*

By simply being concerned — genuinely, of course — about the well-being of others even when our own is not optimal, we exhibit the fundamental attitude of Jesus' own life and mission. Recall for a moment what Our Lord says: "The last will be first and the first will be last" (Matt. 20:16). By placing ourselves in least concern, the Lord will first look upon us in comfort, stability, and consolation. So, it is enough for the Lord that you worry about your family, but pray for them also because even in praying for them (which is truly a great help to them), you also help yourself in both spirit and in body."

Chapter 8:
"Soul-Care"

In chapter 1 of this book, we discussed how much more important the soul is than the body. This, of course, is not guidance or permission to neglect medical treatment or physical care of the body. However, it is vital to realize, accept, remember, and believe that because the soul is what truly makes us "us," we must also care for our souls similar to how we would care for our bodies. In so doing, we also better ourselves in the process. Our bodies would not live, move, or have their being were it not for two supremely important factors: 1) God, and 2) the very soul He gives us. That said, our bodily health is also inextricably connected to our spiritual health, or, the care we give to our souls.

In 1946, an Austrian psychologist, philosopher, and survivor of the Nazi holocaust named Viktor Frankl published a book that would not only become his magnum-opus, but which would also become a staple in the personal libraries of positive-psychologists, mental-health professionals, religious leaders, and spiritual directors throughout the world. A devout adherent to Judaism himself, Frankl believed not only in the soul itself, but also in the immortality thereof, just as Christians do. In fact, Christianity can and proudly does trace its roots back to Judaism in that Jesus, God's only Son and redeemer of all humanity, indeed, God Himself, chose to be incarnated as a Jewish human person, raised in Jewish theology and culture. Judaism, then, should be unashamedly viewed by all Christians as "the older brother of our own faith."

Trained as a psychiatrist, Frankl believed in and subsequently developed a "school of thought" in psychology, well respected, which emphasizes the importance of caring for one's soul, given the reality that, in so doing, one would also care for all other holistic aspects of oneself (i.e.: body, mind, and spirit). His psychological philosophy became known as "logotherapy" which centers around and focuses on "finding meaning and purpose" for the human soul; that is, existence itself, as well as the heartbreaks, joys, pains, sorrows, and triumphs we all experience. His "logotherapy" emphasizes that if human persons can find meaning in their lives, they will have "will-to-live." Relying on his own personal experiences in the Auschwitz death-camp as well as his psychological observations of other innocent prisoners, Frankl posited the principle at the heart of his trademark psychological therapy. According to Frankl, yes, of course, our ultimate quest is to find meaning for our lives as a whole. However, for our purposes, we can take this wholly therapeutic process in "baby-steps."

Rather than focusing on finding meaning and/or purpose for the whole of our lives all at once, we can focus instead on finding meaning from within our immediate struggles with cancer. This is, of course, entirely separate from questioning why we, or anyone, must get, have, or deal with cancer. Frankl is concerned more with facing what we are experiencing head-on, with our soul as a source of strength to carry-on. An example helps. Frankl, in _Man's Search for Meaning_ writes:

> *"Those who have a 'why' to live, can bear with almost any 'how.'"*

Taking at face-value Frankl's wisdom, we must, even if emotionally or physically painful; perhaps intellectually or spiritually exhausting; find a reason to live and to fight through the sometimes agonizing pains of our procedures, chemo rounds, tests, radiation sessions, etc. What can we find from our diagnosis and cancer struggle, in terms of meaning? How will we respond? We have only two real choices: 1) either we can sink so far into despair, fear, and negativity that we lose all of our "will-to-live" or 2) we can find a reason to want to live and in that, then, is found our "meaning;" perhaps not for life as a whole, but at least within our confrontation with cancer. Frank's wisdom and psychological expertise should, I must add, never be seen in any way, as "divorced" from our application to Christian spirituality even though he was Jewish himself. In fact, the monotheism of Judaism as well as the import he places on the soul and the meaning, value, and dignity of human life makes his methods of psychological care **entirely** compatible with Christian spiritual teachings.

In a touching piece of guidance from *Man's Search for Meaning*, Frankl writes:

"Love goes very far beyond the physical person of the beloved. It finds its deepest meaning in his spiritual being, his inner self. Whether or not he is actually present, whether or not he is even still alive at all, ceases to be of importance."

How, given this statement, could we ever possibly doubt Frankl's brilliance in psychology and the "human experience," but more importantly, his faith? Here is a most learned scholar (in Frankl) admitting that love doesn't cease or stop when one we love dies, rejects us, or otherwise distances from us. Love transcends and love endures. As Christians, we, of course, not only believe that God in Jesus Christ is author, perfecter, and Source of Love, but that He is Himself, Love. Therefore, wherever love exists – reciprocated or rejected, embraced or isolated – God is there. St. Paul's words in Hebrews remind us that "Jesus Christ is the same yesterday, today, and forever" (13:8). And if Jesus is God, as we believe, then He is Love, and Love endures… yesterday, today, and forever.

Why, then, ought any of this matter in our cancer struggles? Precisely because Love alone and the endurance; indeed, the permanence thereof gives meaning to not only our struggles, but our entire life. If only Love is what propelled Jesus to endure His own suffering and death for our sake, and that Love for us alone, gave meaning to His life (as well as His suffering), then mustn't Love alone also give meaning to our lives and their sufferings? As we just so recently said, God is present wherever love is because He is Love so, in our struggles with cancer, we ought to hold fast to love as the meaning for which we must seek to love and fight-on. Whether that Love is for our family, our friends, our significant other or spouse, the love of work left to be done or dreams yet to be fulfilled, Scripture reminds us time and again that God, who is Love Himself "is over all and through all and in all" (Ephesians 4:6). To desire to live on for love is to desire what Jesus Himself did, and no matter what, by belief in Him, we share in His destiny: the triumph of Love. In the new preface to Frankl's work, written by bestselling author and rabbi, Harold Kushner, he emphasizes this most valuable point:

"We have come to recognize that this is a profoundly religious book. It insists that life is meaningful and that we must learn to

see it as such despite our circumstances. It emphasizes that there is an ultimate purpose to life."

It's worth adding, of course, that both Jews and Christians believe in "the life of the world to come," and so the meaningfulness or value within this life is inextricably linked to and connected with our "eternal meaning" and our "eternal purpose."

We've spoken, to this point, a good bit about the importance of love providing us with a "will-to-live," and in that vein, though we may wish to "prove our strength" in our cancer struggles, we need to never neglect love or ever think of love as weakness by any means. This doesn't mean just finding our own meaning in love, but it also means allowing ourselves to be loved. And what better "balm for the soul" than someone tenderly expressing their love for us by caring for us when we need it? Perhaps one of the most difficult things about being loved (and thus, "cared for") is the vulnerability that comes with it. A majority of human persons fear such vulnerability because they are afraid of being "caught off-guard" and "hurt." I (and no psychologist or spiritual director "worth their weight") will deny that love certainly carries with it the risk of heartbreak (at least any human love does), but it is also only love that can "heal the soul." Therefore, when the soul has been so "wounded" by the despairs, heartaches, disappointments, or sorrows which inevitably come with a cancer struggle, there is no harm in taking the risk which love demands, especially if, as we have seen, it can heal, renew, and set free.

Earlier, I mentioned that only human love carries with it the weight of risk. This is because God's love is perfect. In His love, there is no risk of disappointment and so, be assured, even if before or in the future, you ever feel "betrayed" by human love, realize that human love carries the risks it does because it is still, no matter how pure, tainted by the stain of sin. I once read a poorly misinformed Tweet which read: "The Bible says "love never fails" so if it fails, just know it was never love." When I first read this, every beat of my heart sank in depression, but not because the Tweet contained _any_ truth-value, but because, as a trained theologian and even more importantly, as a true believer myself, I felt such sorrow for those misled by this person's attempt at what I can only think to call, "drugstore spirituality." I bring this up at this stage in the book because such improper, poorly informed perspectives on such "eternally consequential" matters leads so many astray; and, for our purposes, this is also a fine illustration of why persons are both afraid to be loved or to love others and thus, by extension, are afraid even to be "cared for." The most brilliant theology professor I ever had in both undergraduate and, luckily enough for me, in graduate school as well used to, in all of his courses, emphasize strongly, the importance of context. Contextually, we must be clear on something. When the New Testament was written, it was written in Greek. The passage our surely well-intentioned "Twitter-theologian" referenced was from the New Testament letter of St. Paul to the Corinthians; 1 Corinthians 13:8, just to be clear. The Greek language has <u>four</u> separate words, all with different meanings, for what our English language has as only one.

> ***Eros***: sexual or mere desire; wherefrom the word "erotic" originates.
> ***Storge***: associated with familial affection.
> ***Philia***: "brotherly" love or friendship.
> ***Agape***: selfless, unconditional love; also

understood to be the highest form of
love and the way in which God loves
each of us.

When, in the original Greek, Paul wrote "Love never
fails," what he actually wrote was and is: "God's Love
(*Agape*) never fails." I was pleased to read later that
someone else had commented in response to the initial
Tweet of which I've been referencing; and she did so,
quite eloquently, professionally, and in charity for souls,
correct the incorrectly phrased Tweet. She emphasized,
as is theologically, spiritually, morally, scripturally, and
practically accurate that it is God's love which never
fails. To be crystal-clear, yes, human love can and does
exist which bears also within its presence, God's own.
However, because it is still human, it is still imperfect,
as we are, and thus is capable of failure. Hence, the risk
and vulnerability of love (at least human love) which we
discussed earlier.

This all is worth mentioning as we emphasize
the application of Frankl's logotherapy (through a
Christian lens, of course) as a means of working
through the spiritual and existential questions often
faced by those diagnosed with or undergoing treatment
for cancer. Beyond this, such pivotal information about
the authenticity of love will be useful as we further
discuss the importance of embracing our vulnerability
and allowing ourselves to be helped, cared-for, and yes,
loved when the goings-of-cancer get their toughest. In
the first place, Christian theology admits (and rightly so)
that all human persons are created, foundationally, as
relational-beings. We are made not to live as islands,
but to embrace, choose, and engage actively in love –
including the love for God, family, friends, significant
others, and many times, a combination of these all. In a

moving (yet, still thoroughly psychological, as was his expertise) reflection of how prisoners of the evil Nazi death camps maintained the "will-to-live" even under such brutality, Frankl writes:

> *"The truth – that love is the ultimate and the highest goal to which human persons can aspire" (37).*

Hearing such a statement, for us Christians, may seem almost cliché or trite, however, we mustn't forget the primary identity of God Himself, incarnate in Jesus. Fill in the blanks with me: God Is __ __ __ __. Bearing this in mind, Frankl's next statement is truly a cause for rejoicing! He writes:

> *"The salvation of humanity is through love and in love" (37).*

In the portion of Frankl's *Man's Search for Meaning* entitled, "Logotherapy in a Nutshell," he suggests that within all persons there are at the most basic level, three sources of meaning from which a person can muster the "will-to-live." These, he notes, are:

> 1) For the sake of existence itself,
> 2) For love, and
> 3) In order to obtain dignity through suffering.

I opine, as I'm hopeful also would other theologians, that "the greatest of these is (for) love" (1 Cor. 13:13).

To conclude this chapter on "Soul-Care," I cannot overemphasize the importance of finding within your own soul a reason to keep "fighting-on." Though I may have at times, even recently if we are being honest, questioned my own reasons to "fight on," I cannot deny the brilliance of Frankl's logic and more importantly, the hope, promise, and prize of our Christian faith which is the ultimate Presence, forever, of Love Himself. Time and again, I have been advised by mentors, editors, and even friends never to end a paragraph, paper, or much less a chapter on another person's words. So, while most of these that follow are, in fact, Frankl's, I am ever-so-subtly adapting them with my own. Here, Frankl (and I, in a way), seeks to emphasize all that our souls are capable of, for good purposes. Moreover, since the soul is as immortal as the God who bestowed it upon us, we can be sure that from the past, within the present, or even in the "eternal future," we can find some source from which to draw out that very "will-to-live." Without further ado:

"Whatever you have experienced cannot be taken from you. Not only our experienced, but all we have done, whatever great thoughts we may have had, all we have suffered, [and the love we have had for others,] all this is not lost [for it is immortally part of our soul" (82).

Chapter 9:
"Soul-Friends"

The only aspect of the cancer-struggle more frightening than the diagnosis itself is the potential for day-to-day uncertainty. Perhaps this, on the face of it, sounds quite troubling or even uninspiring, but know that, in the way a good and trusted friend would, I too, am just being honest with you. The beauty of honesty, especially when it comes from a friend, is that they (the good and true ones, at least) have your best interests at heart. So, when I tell you truth from my own experiences that the cancer-struggle can certainly be a frightening one, I do so for your own good... out of honesty, merely to prepare you, not to alarm you. There is another valuable truth which I wish to share with you, out of both Christian friendship and that "special bond," however inexplicable at times, shared by those of us who have ever been "touched" by cancer. The truth is: No matter how frightening the diagnosis or journey through cancer may be, you need not face it alone. True and most importantly, the Good Lord is with us as well as our angel-guardians and the whole Communion of Saints, but God also works in and through people we call "friends." Indeed, in and through our friends, God, in a unique way, is present with us and acting through their love for us, often as other "Simons of Cyrene," who help us carry our crosses just as the original Simon helped Jesus carry His own (cf. Luke 23:26).

Friendship, particularly both the Christian theological and spiritual aspects thereof, has long been an interest of mine, as well as my theological mentor's – this person, who, through our sharing this mutual interest, I am also pleased to call a friend. He pointed out to me on more than one occasion that even the Sacred Scriptures, in both the Old and the New Testaments, praise the importance of friendship. Some examples here include:

From Proverbs:
"A friend loves at all times, and a sibling is born out of their constant love for times of stress" (17:17).

"A true friend is more loyal than a brother" (18:24).

From Sirach:
"A faithful friend is a sturdy shelter; whoever finds one finds a treasure" (6:14).

"A faithful friend can save your life; only those who fear God can know them" (6:16).

From the Gospel of John:
"No one has greater love than to lay down one's life for one's friends" (15:13).

"I no longer call you servants… I call you friends" (15:15).

From Paul's Letter to the Philippians:
"I give thanks to God for you, my friends (1:3).

The scriptural references I have included above are but a few among many throughout the Bible. Some others, though unmentioned here for concision's sake, need not explicitly use the word "friend" outright, but nevertheless speak of the values, qualities, and importance of good friends.

One oft-overlooked (or taken-for-granted) example of such is a three word, one line passage from John's Gospel describing an action of Jesus when He learns that one of his best friends, Lazarus of Bethany, had died. It simply reads:

"And Jesus wept" (11:35).

I find that this short, "one-liner" speaks volumes not only about the importance of genuine friendship to Our Lord, but by extension, what it means for us who are called to the imitation of and devotion to Jesus. Even the Gospel writer, John himself, and every biblical translator, editor, and compiler (no matter which Christian denomination) must also have thought this weeping on the part of Jesus because of His sadness at losing a dear friend was significant. So much so that they gave three words its own line of text and verse number. Let's pay much closer attention, though, especially since this verse is so often overlooked or neglected. Note that it doesn't say "cried" or "shed a tear."

All translating authorities agree that the English conversion from the original Greek out to emphasize something of greater depth and seriousness than mere disappointment, simple sadness, or run-of-the-mill "bad news." To "weep" (the present tense of the past tense "wept") indicates crying and shedding of tears, to be sure, but with deep, nearly piercing pain associated – either of an emotional or physical sort. Weeping is also described as a "nearly inconsolable" form of crying. There is only one other place in the Gospels where Jesus is reported to have "wept" and that was when he overlooked the city of Jerusalem upon His entry into the city (Luke 19:41). This show of emotion was because He knew that this city would reject the One who had literally come to save its people. Surely, we can surmise that Jesus must've cried as a young child when hurt playing or in His agony in Gethsemane, at His scourging, or on the cross, but in these two places only do we learn that Jesus' show-of-emotion far surpassed simple crying. For our purposes, we are only going to continue to treat the first instance related to Lazarus.

Jesus weeps at the news of His friend, Lazarus' passing even knowing He alone possessed the power to resuscitate him because He could not, like so many of us, process what life apart from His friend would be like. In this moving moment in John's Gospel, it is not only the Lord's tears which evidence the depth of Jesus' compassion for Lazarus' sister's sorrow or even His own friendship with Lazarus, but what He does after His weeping. Just as Jesus is the whole embodiment (by the incarnation) of the "eternal Logos," which at creation's dawning "spoke into existence" *ex nihilo*, the incarnate Word speaks a true word of power over the perceived "nothingness" of death. From out of Lazarus' "nothingness-in-death," Jesus calls him forward and though shrouded still, who emerges from the tomb and the "nothingness" of death is not only Lazarus himself, but a living testimony of the value of friendship to the Lord… and hopefully, for us as well. How interesting it is that our only scriptural knowledge of Lazarus is in this portion of John's Gospel! Arguments may be made that Lazarus was a rather obscure or seemingly unimportant New Testament figure, but this seems hard to believe given both that Jesus weeps over his passing and calls him back to life. What this mention of Lazarus more reveals to me is something akin to what a truly brilliant mentor of mine once said to me in an interview we did for our institution's editorial journal. Speaking on the importance of friendship, he said,

"I don't believe God loves us through vague, abstract ideas, but instead in and through the people God has made and situated providentially in our lives" (Scott Geis, "The Galleon," 15 Feb 2017).

Indeed, God does not speak to us only in abstract ideas... He speaks to us best in people. Think, then, of the closest of people He kept around Him, namely, the Apostles. These were "nothing special." In fact, of what we know of the Apostles, they were those whose "merits" (if you would call them such) they most likely would have wanted any excuse to forget. In the best appraisals, their personalities were either "criminal," "crude," or "banal" at best... yet these were whom Jesus called most intimately to love Him, experience Him, and share in His miracles. Hopefully we do, but even if we think our friends are nothing special, we might reconsider in light of the fact that God incarnate placed such value in the perceived "nothingness" of friendship. Quite the contrary, that supposed "nothingness" of friendship meant everything to the Lord... and by His example, it should also to us. I say all of this not only to educate and give hope, but also to assure that as friendship is so esteemed by Jesus Himself, then especially, when we need Him most, namely, in our own confrontation with cancer, we ought not only cling to Him, but the sorts of things He values... chief among them, friendship.

In Celtic (or generally Irish) early Christianity, from the times of Sts. Brigid and Patrick, a unique and beautiful spiritual expression emerged related to friendship. In the midst of a personal confrontation with cancer, one will often find themselves engaging introspectively with their own interior and sometimes "most hidden" thoughts; more so, likely one may incline to examine the health of their soul… or lack thereof. The physical burdens associated with any cancer struggle are, quite naturally, daunting enough, although it is generally routine in the human condition for persons to also become more interiorly reflective when confronted with suffering. To have to face both physical suffering in addition to emotio-spiritual suffering apart from the comfort of another person is among the more intensely negative circumstances. Fortunately, early Irish Christians, recognizing this "long loneliness" as well as God's own Words that "it is not good for humanity to be alone" (Gn. 2:18), gave first words to a spiritual principle still valued throughout the Christian world today. This Celtic Christian spiritual concept is known as **anamchara**. In Gaelic, the word "anam" means "soul" and "chara," "friend." Together, the Celtic Christians developed the spirituality of *soul-friends*.

The term, "soul-friend" may well often bring into mind the similarly titled and oft-overused term, "soul-mate." But rest assured, there is a difference between the two, neither of which most persons have ever likely investigated. To be sure, a "soul-mate" is generally understood as a person with whom you have an instantaneous "connection" either romantically or in friendship upon meeting the person. The common misconception among the majority of the population is that one's "soul-mate" is only ever "romantic" in nature. Not so. Furthermore, a "soul-mate" is often proclaimed to be so by one or both parties from an early stage in the relationship when the person or persons have not come to know the "eternally intimate" details of one another's lives. In this way, the term "soul-mate" is somewhat superficial at best. Conversely, and much more positively, a "soul-friend" (anamchara) is understood as "being joined in both an ancient and eternal way with the 'friend of your soul.'" The Irish writer, John O'Donohue, provides us with that understanding. Further, we should note that one's "soul-friend" need not only be one's "friend" in the Platonic sense although this is also certainly acceptable. The "soul-friend" concept is similar, spiritually and theologically, to St. Aelred of Riveaulx's explanation and discourse on "spiritual friendship." A simple Google search will yield more insight into this. Ultimately, "soul-friends" very much unlike "soul-mates," are anything superficial. "Soul-friends" know a person sometimes even more intimately than they know themselves. Beyond this, one's "soul-friend" often acts as a confidante, companion, spiritual mentor, and personal confessor.

All that said, we need not carry our burdens throughout life, or especially in our confrontation with cancer, alone. Certainly, we have God's ever-abiding Presence, but perhaps also, we might do well to lean on our "soul-friends;" they who are, after all, God's gifts of Himself to us. "Soul-friends" can be, to us, persons we have known for years (either family or friends), but can also be someone we meet as we undergo treatment for cancer. These persons; namely, those we befriend through treatment, may connect with us at first simply because of a share in a similar adversity, but over time, we may begin to glimpse within them elements truly spiritual, eternal, and profound in friendship. To bring this chapter to conclusion, I wish to end with three brief, but valuable observations:

1) St. Aelred of Riveaulx wrote an entire book on the importance of friendship in the Christian spiritual life in the 12th century simply titled, *Spiritual*

Friendship. He insists that authentic "soul-friends" exist in a tripartite relationship. He writes, "Here we are, you and I, and I hope, a third, Christ, is in our midst. If "God is Love" as we acknowledge Him to be, and friendship is a form of love (Philia) [for more, see *The Four Loves* by C.S. Lewis], then it stands, as Aelred argues, that God is truly an ever-present third-party in the love of friendship; a Presence most important who even acts as "the glue" or solidifying element in such friendships. Through our friends, we find yet another way in which God Himself is present with us as we carry "the cross of cancer."

2) Friends, especially in the "cancer-journey," can provide a support system which, for the patient, we may particularly crave and that is beyond our families or spouses. We might crave the uniqueness of a friend-based support system because perhaps they can internalize both good and bad news better than can our families or spouses. If your family is anything like mine was during my struggle, then they either "over-expect" good news or "profusely lament" bad news. There was no "in-between," but friends can be this "in-between" and in many ways, that level-headedness can keep us sane and be further conducive to our healing. Perhaps also, friends may provide the much-needed socialization amidst the sometimes inevitable isolation of the "cancer-journey." When the chemo or radiation decimates our immune systems and we can seldom see or visit with others, we feel the height of cancer's mercilessly isolative capabilities, but friends will be who you can call, Skype, text, or write letters to (yes, a select few of us still do the latter); all of which comforts and allows us to recall that we aren't alone in our struggle.

3) Last, but certainly not least: Our friends will pray for us; and we ought to pray for them as well. In

my experience, close friends become family such that our own family comes to know them and theirs, us. That interchange necessarily includes in "the willful obligations of friendship," prayer for one another.

Chapter 10:
Cross of a Different Kind

"Take up your cross, the Savior said,
If you would my disciple be; deny yourself,
Forsake the world, and humbly follow after me."
~ From a hymn by Charles Everest

As you've likely already noticed, the title of this chapter is, in itself, the name-source of the entire book. While I certainly believe the chapters that precede this one as well as those that follow after it are all equally important in their own ways, this chapter, though situated in the section of this book that particularly addresses those currently fighting the battle against cancer, is one from which the contents are applicable to all groups addressed throughout this text.

In Christian theological circles, primarily in the halls of academia, there generally emerge two "believing-camps." While neither side stands any way in contradiction or opposition to the other, the focus of each theological camp can certainly be evident not only in writing, but also in perspective. These two "believing-camps" in Christianity concern the single event in the life of Christ considered most significant to the particular theologian and believer. Perhaps unknown to many of us, whether formally educated in theology or not makes no difference as each one of us, in belief, spirituality, and personal relationship with the Divine, tend to "sway" towards one "believing camp" more so than another.

One perspectival side holds that the Crucifixion and sacrificial death of Jesus was the most pivotal event in His life and, as a result, is the most significant event for those of us who believe in, hope in, and adore Him to focus on in our spiritual lives. As you may have rightly assumed, the other of the two perspectival sides looks to the Resurrection of Jesus as His exalted life's most pivotal event, thus deriving from it spiritual focus for the lives of believers. To put all of this more succinctly, I've found one of the best explanations in a very wise and trusted duo of colleagues of mine who framed these perspectival differences thusly:

> "…*There are two ways of thinking about God in Christ. These two ways encompass the whole breadth of human experience and salvation… a "theologia gloriae" (theology of glory, the Risen Christ) that points to joy and a "theologia crucis" (theology of the Cross, the Crucified Christ) that emphasizes suffering, humility, dependence, and vulnerability"* (Watson & Parker, *Sports, Religion, & Disability*, p. 5).

Purposely, I mention these perspectival differences at the outset of this chapter in order to dispel any thought that one perspective is any more important or valid than any other, at least in this context. In reality and Divine Truth, the Passion, Death, and Resurrection of Jesus, while indeed three separate events of _human_ history, are, in fact, all part of one event in the far more crucial _salvation_ history. For this reason, the Church universal upon opening the Holy Week celebration of The Lord's Supper on Holy (or Maundy) Thursday, does not conclude the celebration until the close and dismissal of the Easter Vigil during the Easter Triduum. The three events – Passion, Death, and Resurrection of Christ – then, are all part of one salvific act of love on our behalf. All that said, and keeping in mind that, on the whole, focus on either the Crucifixion or the Resurrection ought never be to the diminution of one's importance to the other, there are times in the spiritual journey wherein it may be helpful to meditate more intently on the meaning and ontological impact of either the Crucifixion or the Resurrection of Jesus.

The personal confrontation with the displeasures (to put it mildly) of cancer present us with one such opportunity to, perhaps more intently than we already do, reflect on the mysteries and significance of Jesus' Crucifixion. Well before Jesus' own way of "practicing what He preached" (in a most literal sense), He said to His Apostles, and thus, to all of us as well:

"Whoever wishes to come after me must deny himself, take up his cross, and follow me. For whoever wishes to save his life will lose it, but whoever loses his life for my sake will save it"
(Matt 16:24-25).

It is important to realize that this is advice for spiritual maturity from a most reliable Source, but also that our Source, Jesus Himself, doesn't simply tell His followers to do this, never to return to it Himself. Quite literally, Jesus leads by example. Without doubt, He denies Himself by submitting not to His own will (see Matthew 26:42), but to that of God, His (and our) Father with whom He has always and still shares filial communion. He quite obviously and literally took up His cross and followed His own exhortation in laying down His life. In the process, He saves His own life as evidenced by the Resurrection. Not only does Jesus save His own life in willful obedience, but ours in the process. The cross was and is of paramount importance to Jesus, so much so that He even speaks of it in the Gospels a full ten chapters before He is ever sentenced to carry His own! Aside from a mere reminder of the boundless depths of Jesus' love for each of us as well as a sign of victory over death, sin, sorrow, humiliation, pain, suffering, and shame, the Cross in the Christian spiritual life remains a means of hope-fulfilled for those of us who suffer physically, or in any other way, particularly for our purposes, in the confrontation with cancer, in any of its wicked forms.

Since, in our largely Western society and culture, crucifixion is no longer an execution method, the meaning and applicable nature of Jesus' Words in Matthew 16:24 are often questioned. *What must it mean for me to "take up my cross" in the 21st century?* A "cross" is merely a suffering-laced burden of some sort; and true enough, we all have those, don't we? For those suffering with cancer, the identity of "the Christ in agony," trudging along in excruciating pain under the weight of the heavy cross-beams, is often most profound and relatable. While it's true that in Jesus' suffering, He took on all sins past, present, and future of all humanity therefore making His own suffering (and the subsequent victory over it, I should note) far greater than anything any of us could ever experience, it is also true that the agonies and rarities of cancer are also far greater than the average suffering experiences of the general population. Because of this, a cancer patient looking at the face of Christ on the cross in a religious painting, icon, or other depiction is likely more apt to not only notice the agony and sorrow on His holy face, but to also think something akin to the idea, "Same, Lord. Me too;" this of course, an expression of mutual unity in agony and suffering. In this way, namely because cancer and its associated treatments often cause suffering, cancer can be truly viewed as a "cross" and most surely at that, one of "a different kind," indeed.

In the confrontation with cancer, there also is the dimension of a fundamental change to one's quality of life – at least for a time, if not permanently, to some degree. This is significant because Jesus also talks about those seeking to save their lives and those who will lose them. Certainly, the all-loving (Omni-Benevolent) God in Jesus Christ does not wish for a person who takes up their own cross and follows Him to perish needlessly or to perish as a choice merely to avoid suffering. In context of the confrontation with cancer, Jesus' Words take on a practical meaning. When cancer comes, it takes from us a certain quality of life as long as we have it. The treatments to combat and hopefully defeat it also diminish at times the qualities of life we have, prior to diagnosis, grown so accustomed to as well. By embracing the "cross of cancer," as Jesus carrying so embraced His own "cross of wood," we already are making the choice to, in a literal sense, "lay down our life," as we have come to know it. And the hard truth of the matter is that even in survival, life after cancer (and certainly while during) is never again quite the same. This is by no means meant to arouse distress or sadness within you, but to encourage you, believe it or not. For in embracing our cross, we too, like the Lord, shall save our eternal life, even by means of enduring the physical sufferings of this life.

In terms of our physical life, the suffering we face in cancer takes on an ontologically different purpose itself. While Christian theology holds that the existence of suffering in the world is as a result of humanity's "fall" into sin and from the "state-of-grace," we ought never to think of ourselves as being punished by God through our sufferings. This would make of God more a "monster" than a "lover." God does not, I repeat, punish us through our sufferings. In fact, the

God of Christianity that is the One, True God, incarnate in His very Son, Jesus, loves all His human creation to such excess that He – that is, God Himself – chose not only to redeem suffering, as a distinctly human experience, but to embrace it so as to fully share in and utterly empathize with us when we suffer. This is contained in the mystery, significance, and power of the Cross. When hanging on the cross in agony, Jesus experienced the worst evils of humanity, in a truly personal sense, such that He even succumb – for a time – to the point of death as a result of the horrific nature of those evils. "Deicide" is the distinctly theological term which refers to "the murder of the Divine Being." For Christians, obviously, this is God in the Person of Jesus Christ. To say that Jesus died to redeem all humankind from our sinfulness is entirely true and valid, but it also doesn't go nearly far enough. Instead, it should be clear that Jesus died _because_ of our sins. This means, in the most unnerving and stark of ways, all humankind, complicit in collective and personal sinfulness, are co-committers of "deicide." This is worth mentioning in order to thoroughly comprehend the depths of Jesus' salvific action. Indeed, Jesus so loves His human creation – each one of us as if we were His only love – at so great a depth that though we murdered Him by our sins, He chooses still to redeem us and love us in spite of such horror. Now consider this: while it is true that Jesus took into Himself and destroyed all human sinfulness by suffering the greatest and worst of all evils and pains to which there can be no comparison, should this mean that we, Jesus' own creation, should no longer suffer in this life?

To appropriately answer this question, we must first remember that Jesus, though always Divine in nature as God Himself, was also simultaneously entirely human. Jesus was and is, truly, "one like us in all things but sin." If even God Himself shared in the sufferings of this physical life and body, then how much more so should we suffer? After all, we are not superiors to God. The fact that we suffer, however, need not ever be viewed as mere vanity. Perhaps I should say, "Need not *any longer* be viewed as mere vanity." Having embraced, personally experienced, and overcome suffering Himself, Jesus redeemed and sanctified suffering single-handedly by the greatest of all attributes: Love. Were it not for love of each one of us, perfect obedience to the Father's will that humanity be restored to friendship with Himself in His Son would also not have been a possibility. The evidence that Jesus has given a noble and redeeming nature to suffering exists in the fact that God the Father raises Him from death to life again in the splendor of the Resurrection. Upon rising from certain death, the Gospels narrate in several instances, that Jesus still bears the now indelible marks of His suffering. Were these wounds – clear and obvious reminders of suffering – irrelevant, they would cease to have existed as part of the Christ's glorified, Risen, and restored corpus. That even in His Resurrection, Jesus bears the hands, feet, and side wounds of His Passion shows outwardly that He has redeemed and conquered over the evils of suffering, opening to all who believe in Him not only hope that they, like He in whom they believe, can conquer over such evils, but that by uniting their sufferings with those of suffering's first conqueror, they also may share in the very redemption purchased by Jesus Christ in the endurance of such sufferings. This is of valuable importance, especially to those suffering the confrontation with cancer. By uniting the agonies, pains, humiliations, and sorrows of the cancer experience with those same agonies, pains, humiliations, and sorrows experienced by the Lord Himself for our own sake, our own sufferings, by the power of Jesus' Passion, become sanctified, made holy. To that end, since our sufferings – only, mind you, when intentionally united to Christ's by the action of prayerful offering – are holy, they can also be utilized as a means of prayer themselves when, in our own weaknesses, we simply cannot find the right words. Through these "prayers of suffering," we can and do "pray without ceasing" (1 Thessalonians 5:16) even when, in the midst of our own physical pain, emotional turbulence, intellectual fogginess, or spiritual dryness, we find it difficult to engage in more traditional methods of prayer.

There is yet another aspect of Jesus' suffering worth our reflection when considering our own. How often, amidst intense pain or sadness, do we become doubtful of God's ever-abiding and continuously loving Presence? I'll be the first to admit that there have been (and are) times when I feel almost "abandoned" by God in my own pains, sadness, or struggles. In those moments of weakness, we are anything but abandoned. In fact, in our weakest moments, Jesus could not be any closer to us than were we to be standing in the radiance of the Beatific Vision. Do you remember Jesus' own lament from the cross? "My God! My God, why have you abandoned me?!" (Matthew 27:46), Jesus cried out in excruciating pain! Skeptics quickly point to this verse in attempts to make the claim that Jesus Himself is not "very God of very God." However, Truth requires, and thus provides, a much more compelling response. In the very moment when Jesus questions the nearness of His Father, God's silent yet powerfully certain answer was within Jesus' very self. Very God of Very God had not at all abandoned His Son – not in the slightest. In reality, because Jesus is fully God Himself, Jesus' own lament points to the absolutely remarkable depth of loving intervention. The Creator, Redeemer, and King of all creation that ever was, is, or will be, had in the moment of Jesus' cry from the cross, left the Heavenly throne and was, Himself, there present in the triumphant and conquering suffering of His only Son and very self. God quite literally could not have been any closer to Jesus in that moment. This is comfort for those of us who believe in Jesus. We can be sure that when we suffer and wonder about God's proximity to us that He is, in the slightly modified words of Saint Augustine, "more interior to us than we are to ourselves."

Earlier in this chapter, we spoke briefly about the portion of Jesus' exhortation in Matthew 16:24 which speaks of denying one's self. In my experiences in chaplaincy with teen cancer patients and their parents, the idea of continuing the ancient Christian spiritual practice of self-denial (also known as "asceticism") at all, much less during the trials of cancer, is often met, at least at first, with certain consternation. Understandably so, however, I have witnessed first-hand the spiritually valuable benefits of the practice of self-denial even while having to carry this "cross of a different kind." The usual thought-process surrounding self-denial during the cancer experience often operates based around the idea that cancer already takes so many liberties from us and forces us into having to live without certain aspects of life we may enjoy (e.g.: energy, appetite, sex-drive, physical strength, etc.) and increases, almost just as forcefully, aspects of life we don't enjoy (e.g.: isolation from friends, physical limitations, increased anxieties, etc.). Therefore, if already forced by so sinister an illness to be denied of as many joyful aspects of life, why should anyone willingly choose to deny themselves anything more than they already have to? Admittedly, this is a brilliant question and when I first encountered it from a wise-beyond-her-years 17 year old cancer patient, I was without an answer for her. Several weeks went by before I saw this brave young lady again, but when I did, she had the best demeanor about her (as well as one could in a hospital for chemotherapy rounds) as well as an answer to her own question that reduced me to tears of joyfully simplistic profundity, as well as stunned silence. To say that I was taught that day by someone I was in some way responsible for teaching, or at least guiding, would be an understatement. She went far beyond merely teaching me an answer to her original question which stumped me. She "lived the answer" into existence.

When I entered her room that afternoon to give her the Eucharist and a blessing, I found her experiencing the typical chemotherapy-associated nausea; so much so that she excused herself for a moment from my presence to throw-up in hopes that if she "got it out of the way," she could receive the Eucharist without also throwing it back up. Emerging from the restroom, she declined the Sacrament that day, but asked instead if she could simply receive a blessing. Understanding her wishes, I happily obliged. After praying over and with her, she asked if I had a few moments to talk while her mother was attempting to get some much needed sleep in the adjoining parent-room. I agreed. Without missing a beat, she said, "Remember last time you saw me and I asked you about why I should have to give up any more than what the tumor has already made me?" Amazed myself that she remembered or would even care, I said, "I do and I think..." She stopped me. "I think I've figured it out... well, for me, at least," she said. Here were her stunning words: "So, its Lent and you mentioned that self-denial stuff. I guess I could at least try to deny myself the satisfaction of being a jerk about all this. I mean, it's nobody's fault. Nobody gave me cancer. Sometimes it may be hard for me to want to smile, like when you heard me throwing-up earlier. I was embarrassed and could have asked you to leave. I still don't feel great, but here we are." I still remember those words of hers just as clearly as I write this down today as if she had just spoken them to me. When I left her room that day, they lingered with me too. Her attitude and outlook changed me and my entire ministerial approach for the better. I am so grateful to have encountered this patient; and all my patients for that matter. Uplifting anecdotes aside, the wisdom of her answer is everywhere rooted in spiritual truth. Often times, in the Christian spiritual life, we mistakenly assume that self-denial necessarily means giving something up rather than doing some other positive act. In their wonderful handbook on Christian spirituality, Lawrence Cunningham and Keith Egan write:

"For a person to be a follower of Jesus it becomes necessary to say "no" to certain ways of thinking acting, or being" (Christian Spirituality, pg. 110).

While cancer can sometimes make us feel bitter, mean-spirited, or even resentful, we still possess the power of choice to say "no" to these emotions. That sort of "no" can not only free us from being hurtful to those who are usually only trying to be helpful to us in comfort amidst treatment, but it also frees us to replace and enjoy contentment over resentment, kind-heartedness over mean-spiritedness, and cheerfulness over bitterness. These attitudes, in the process, will likely help to cultivate not only more joy in the midst of suffering, but also a deeper and more fruitful spiritual maturity.

To this point, we've spoken much of the value of both denying ourselves and taking up that "cross of a different kind" that is cancer, but like Jesus' own history, there is life beyond the Cross. Certainly, our journey through the cancer experience will be a struggle, but Jesus' own confrontation with and harrowing of suffering gives all of us, His children, hope and blessed assurance that, by His Divine assistance, we too, may overcome such suffering, having attained from it greater appreciation for the depths to which we are loved and thus, compelled to love. Through the sufferings of our own crosses, we become further fashioned into images of Christ, able then to outwardly reflect to all we encounter, the promise of triumph over suffering through He who is both Resurrection and Life.

Suggested Spiritual Exercises & Further Resources
Part II

1) Christianity is by no means a "passive" way-of-life; quite the contrary, in fact. The beliefs in and about Jesus Christ which we profess call us to "active engagement." One such activity in which we all must actively engage in the spiritual life is the battle of "spiritual warfare," or the ongoing pursuit of the prevailing of goodness over evil.

   - *Take some time to make a list of ways in which you feel that "the powers of darkness" are attempting to "entrap" you through your confrontation with cancer; then devise your own unique spiritual "battle plan" through which you can and will fight against and overcome the darkness of hopelessness.*

2) Admire your "battle scars."

   - *When I have suggested this spiritual technique in the past to groups, it has always been met with some surprise. Some may think it to be a bit morbid, but hey, wounds are "kind of a big deal" for Christians. So, yes, admire your own bruises, scars, surgical incisions, etc. that you have obtained through your own battle with cancer. When admiring them, do so with remembrance of Jesus' own "battle scars," His Holy Wounds in mind, and know that His scars have made yours truly beautiful!*

3) Consider obtaining a larger printed copy of the poem entitled, *What Cancer Cannot Do*. The author of this poem remains unknown, but its truth-value is undeniable. For your own reference, a copy of this poem is provided below:

What Cancer Cannot Do

It cannot cripple Love

It cannot shatter Hope

It cannot corrode Faith

It cannot destroy Peace

It cannot kill Friendship

It cannot suppress Memories

It cannot silence Courage

It cannot invade the Soul

It cannot steal Eternal Life

It cannot conquer the Spirit.

-Author Unknown

4) The multi-dimensional pains of cancer and associated treatments can sometimes plunge us nearly into the depths of despair such that we may at times be tempted to just "give-up." **Don't!**

    - Identify three facets / aspects / things for which you wish to continue living. Write these down and keep them always near you. Allow them to motivate you as they remind you that you have the "will-to-live!"

5) Spend time with and confide in your friends.

    - Allow yourself to be vulnerable around them; lay bare your soul to them, acknowledging that Christ's Spirit is ever present in friendship.

- Write a letter to someone you consider to be your "soul-friend(s) and make sure you make clear how much you love, value, and appreciate them. This will make them happy as well as you in the process.

6) Practice self-denial.
- Deny yourself the opportunities for bitterness, meanness, or resentment and attempt to practice cheerfulness, kindness, and gentleness.

7) Consider reading:
- <u>*Man's Search for Meaning*</u> *by Viktor Frankl*
- <u>*Salvivici Doloris*</u> *by Pope St. John Paul II*
- <u>*Meditations on the Cross*</u> *by Dietrich Bonhoeffer*

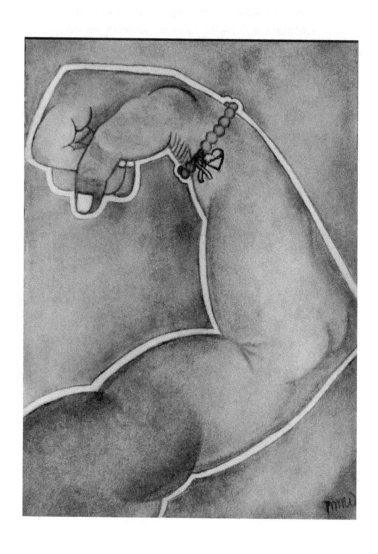

© Mirjana Walther, 2017

Part III

The Fullness of Life

"For Cancer Survivors"

Chapter 11:
Physical (βίος) and Spiritual (ζωή) Life

At the outset of any survivor-spirituality, we would be entirely remiss if we did not first acknowledge that survivorship in cancer is never achievable apart from God's grace, chiefly and to be sure. Then, in addition, the numerous intercessory prayers offered on our behalf by friends, acquaintances, and loved-ones as well as the Holy Spirit's role in calling our doctors, nurses, and other medical healthcare personnel to their respective healing vocations. Moreover, we wholly miss the point of any constructive survivor-spirituality the moment we fail to remember our sisters and brothers who have gone to their eternal rest as a result of cancer. All of these persons – that includes, in order: God, our departed cancer-family, all who prayed for us during our confrontation with the illness, and our medical treatment teams – are those upon whose backs we safely traversed the often violent and stormy seas of the cancer journey. For them all, not only should we be especially grateful, but, in a very real way, just as the Apostles devoted their lives in imitation of and devotion to Jesus because of their gratitude for His sacrifice of love, we also, out of gratitude for the sacrifices made by others that we may stand among those called "survivors," ought to imitate their selflessness, generosity, and thoughtfulness.

As cancer-survivors, we have been given a unique perspective as to the value of using both our physical and spiritual lives not only as means through which to relate personally to God in Jesus Christ, but also to more deeply understand the complexities and intricacies of what it means to be human. This somewhat heightened awareness of our own humanity is also valuable in that it aids in the constructive cultivation of relationships with others who so obviously share in our human complexity. Stated quite bluntly, those of us who have faced-down cancer have been to death's doorstep and all but crossed the threshold. To prolong the metaphor, we have peered through the frosted windows of that door and have come away renewed with a zest-for-life and a desire to live life to its fullest, glorifying the Lord by our lives, and certain in the hope of eternal life to come. To live in this renewed sense of the "fullness of life" does not mean living carelessly or with a sort of reckless-abandon, but in a dynamic unity of both body and soul. While it remains true as ever that the body is eventually subject to decline and decay and that the soul remains immortally unchanged, Christians do not view the body or the soul as being in any way in contrast or competition with one another (lest we fall into the heretical ideas of Gnosticism). Instead, as Christians, we reverence the value of the body as a vessel through which, animated by the soul, we may praise God through our good works. For greater clarity, we turn to both the originality and authenticity of the Christian scriptures.

Greek was the original language in which the New Testament (the Gospels, Acts of the Apostles, Pauline Epistles, further letters, and Revelation) was written. Rather than Hebrew (in which the Old Testament was written) or Aramaic (as Jesus and the Apostles would have spoken conversationally), Greek was likely chosen because it was a more widely known trade-acquired language and therefore, the accessibility to the scriptures would also have met a much broader audience. That said, the Greek language is far more precise than our English one. This is relevant on more than one occasion when it comes to understanding the true meanings and contexts of many portions of scripture. For our purposes – namely, endeavoring to understand the renewed emphasis and value of life for cancer-survivors – we will take up the specificity and differences in reality, utilizing the original Greek, for the word we simply know as "life."

In English, like the word "love," we have but one "catch-all" term for "life," but this is not the case in Greek, the original language of the New Testament. In fact, the word "life" has two meanings in Greek. Depending on context, the word "bios" (βίος) (the root from which we get the term, "biology") refers specifically to "physical" or "embodied" life. References to this particular use of the word would often be made only when discussing the material components necessary for "physical life" such as blood, flesh, breath, etc. The second Greek term used is "zóé" (ζωή), which literally translates to mean, "fullness of life," or even "spirit-filled life," from which we derive the term, "spiritual life." Interestingly enough, even early semi-pagan Greeks believed in the immortality of the soul and even believed that a body could not be "fully alive" (zóé) unless such a body was animated by the soul. I suppose even the pagans got one right every now and then. But, I digress: There are, in John's Gospel, Words from Jesus which are, of course, applicable to us all, but which may take on special meaning for the cancer-survivor, in particular. In the tenth chapter, Jesus says,

"I came that you may have life, and have it in abundance"
(Jn. 10:10).

Used in this verse, in its original Greek, is the form zóé, meaning just as translated, "fullness of life," "life in abundance," and/or "spiritual life." All translations are equivalent or can be used interchangeably.

What Jesus does here in saying this is really quite remarkable. Effectively, He discourages mediocrity. Jesus doesn't merely want us to enjoy life as if though only bound to our bodies. If that were the case, oh how limited we all would be, even those who have been entirely healthy their entire lives. If only we could live and enjoy life through bodily means, all of our existence would be utterly fleeting, temporary, and quite lackluster as we'd only ever be chasing after our next pleasurable moment. However, because Jesus has come, embraced a body like ours, and through that body, personally confronted and conquered evil, sin, sadness, and death, He has redeemed the body such that what we experience through life in the body in joy may be retained through the immortality of life in the Spirit! Take, for example, someone we dearly came to love in this life. We came to know them through the medium of the body, but even should they be physically or emotionally lost to us, our memories of them and love for them endure eternally within our souls.

To assert that zóé (our spiritual life) makes all life worth living, and joyfully so at that, would be quite the understatement. It is, in fact, only by life in the Spirit that we physically live (βίος) at all. Elsewhere in John's Gospel, Jesus says,

"I am the Way, the Truth, and the Life" (Jn. 14:6).

Even here, the Greek used for life is zóé, making clear this importance of "Divine Wholeness." Moreover, Jesus' Words there in John 14:6 may be read another way: *"I am the Way **who is** the Truth **which leads to** the **fullness of** Life."* Jesus goes on just after saying this to say, "No one comes to the Father except through" Him. This is so significant because Jesus' own Words contain within them promises. All that we experience in this life is not in vain, whether sorrowful or joyful, painful or peaceful. Through Jesus, we enter into the Father, to live everlasting where all is made new. Indeed, in the Divine Love that is zóé, this fullness of life everlasting, every joyous or happy moment from this life is more than magnified; every sorrowful or sad moment erased from memory and replaced instead by the inexhaustible mercy of Divine Comfort.

Jesus' Words from the Gospels truly are to us "good news!" There is abundant freedom in the knowledge that Jesus desires for us to enjoy our lives and to live in the fullness of His Spirit. Even if our own battle with cancer has left us "wounded" in the physical body (bios), Jesus' Words about ushering in the fullness of life (zóé) are just as relevant, including for traumatic emotional wounds as well. Living with a renewed vision of the fullness of life demands of us a radically new way of living. Remember, we have been close to that veil between life and death so now that we live in the dawn of our "new life" on the other side of cancer, we ought to seek opportunities – again, even if physically or emotionally scarred by our battle – to live that "abundant life" unhindered by the fear of death, pain, or infirmity, which so long plagued us. Consider all the Apostles, once more: their lives before following Jesus were rough to say the least, but Jesus willed that they not be defined by their old lives. Our confrontation with cancer will always be part of our own story just as the Apostles' lives before Jesus will always be part of theirs, but the point here is that our life with cancer need not define us. In more ways than one, Jesus has given us newness of life. The question for us then becomes: *"Thankful for this renewed life, how will I glorify God and help His people in the process by living it?"*

Chapter 12:
A Life Not Our Own

In our previous chapter, we spoke a bit about not simply life itself, but the "abundant life," "the fullness of life," or what we might call "a life imbued by the Spirit" (all appropriate understandings of the Greek word ζωή). The cancer-survivor develops, generally, a "new-lease-on-life," if you'll pardon the old idiom, in having confronted a life-threatening illness. For most, the confrontation with such does more than simply make one mindful of one's own mortality. In a very real way, the endurance of the illness and the realization that one's illness has entered remission presents a poignant juxtaposition whereby awareness of mortality meets and very nearly touches awareness of morality, or the extents to which certain ways of living are either right or wrong. Christian theology teaches that the actions of those of us who are adherents to the teachings of Jesus Christ act rightly (or morally) when we imitate and devote ourselves to the sorts of actions valued by God-incarnate in Jesus Himself, and as revealed to us by means of sacred scripture and sacred tradition. Surviving a catastrophic illness like cancer certainly presents us with opportunities to evaluate our own ways of living and to then, informed by the insights gleaned from our evaluation, determine how to best take advantage of that "new-lease-on-life" we've been given in the hopes of experiencing in this earthly life some share in that very "fullness of life" (zóé) that we hope to attain eternally in the life to come. Cynthia Siegfried, in her remarkable book, *Cancer Journey*, puts it this way:

"Illness is transformative. You will be changed, and in the hands of God those changes can be positive. Your journey... can give birth to increased creativity" (pg. 121).

As Christians, we believe that the Holy Spirit is the Source of both inspiration and creativity so in the midst of the changes we may have experienced in our own cancer struggles, it has ever been the Holy Spirit who lovingly points us into deeper reflection as to how the ways in which we live (morality) can and will impact our quality-of-life here on earth (mortality) as well as the eternal life of the world to come.

Though secularly Jewish and likely spiritually agnostic, it was the famed scientist, Albert Einstein, who said:

"Only a life lived for others is a life well-lived."

His quote and the wisdom it contains are wholly supported by Christian morality. God, in His infinite wisdom, not only created each one of us in His own image and likeness, but also as beings made for relationship. This very reality is also contained in the mysteriousness, but no less valid, doctrine of the Holy Trinity. God Himself dwells and exists eternally in an inexhaustible exchange of love and communion, united as One, in the Father (the Source of Creation), the Son (the Source of Redemption), and the Holy Spirit (the Source of Inspiration). Since human beings, each of us and equally, are created in the very image of God who is Himself a Trinity, and thus actively engaged in relationship, it follows logically that we too, are made for active engagement in relationships. None of us can live and thrive successfully alone. All this considered, it also bears mentioning that any constructive spirituality necessarily exists in a unity of relationship from out of which one's self actively engages with both God and others. If this is true, as we believe in Christianity, then we also must, even if begrudgingly at first, come to acknowledge the truth that this life (including even our second-chance as survivors) is **_not_** our own. Some caveats before proceeding to explain:

    1) Yes, we have free-will and can choose to act and live as we wish. However, certain choices which are pleasing to God allow us to more richly experience the "fullness of life," not only in this life, but in the eternal one.

    2) The realization that our lives are not our own finds root and authenticity in Jesus' own life and example. His entire life was lived as a sacrifice for the sake of others (including each one of us personally) and in obedience to the will of His Father. Therefore, since we are made in the image of One whose life was not His own, neither then is ours our own to live selfishly.

What all of this means for cancer-survivors is really quite simple. We have, placed upon our lives by the very virtue of the fact that we are survivors, a calling from God! Indeed, we are called to be lights to others who, in any ways, find themselves thrust into the darkness of confrontation with the evils of cancer. God has chosen us to, as St. Benedict of Nursia once wrote:

"Go to help the troubled and be of consolation to those in any sorrow" (Rule, 4:18-19).

We, as survivors, have a unique position, opportunity, obligation, and skill-set by which to answer such a call. Simultaneously, we serve and honor God by helping our fellow human beings created in His own image. We can do all of this in several ways which include, but are not limited to:

1) Using our stories of survival to encourage and give hope to others still fighting cancer.

2) Remaining involved, as advocates, in both cancer survivorship and in advancement of support for cancer research.

3) By embracing (and not suppressing) the memories and experiences of our own cancer struggle.

4) Being mindful of the persons who helped us along throughout our own journey through cancer as well as those who have "gone before us."

5 Never neglecting to care for ourselves by getting regular check-ups and screenings; and by participating in research, as possible.

Each of these ways are means of "giving back" to a unique and dynamic community to which we all now belong as cancer-survivors. For the remainder of this chapter, we will take each of the aforementioned ways of "giving back" in turn and examine their spiritual as well as practical values in hopes of coming to the realization that each of us truly can (and is called to) help one another carry this "cross of a different kind."

The first of five ways cancer-survivors can both be of valuable help and "give back" in gratitude for life to the cancer-community is through using our own stories and experiences with our own cancer struggles to positively help and uplift others still engaged in their own fight. To be sure, we ought not brag in any way about our survival to those still endeavoring to become what we are or to those who have lost loved-ones to it lest we do more emotional and spiritual harm than good. Instead, what our experiences offer us are the abilities to empathize with those who are suffering and to, in a very real way, "walk with them" as companions. Others who are actively confronting cancer diagnoses or treatments enter into their experiences just as we did: with fear of what is to come in the journey, doubts about the efficacy of treatment, and sometimes, even a palpable despair or loneliness brought on by the concern that no one will understand their adversities. As persons who have been through the cancer-gauntlet before and have come out alive on the other side, we have knowledge we can share with others just beginning such an arduous journey. Not only do we have this knowledge, we have a moral responsibility to help these sisters and brothers of ours.

Recall the Words of Jesus in Matthew's Gospel: *"Whatever you do for the least of my people, this you do to me"* *(25:40)*. We might also read, in this context, seeing in fellow cancer-sufferers the image of the agonized Christ in Gethsemane, *"Whatever we do not do for the least of God's people, that we do not do to Him."* Who among us, now blessed with another chance to live the fullness of life on the other side of cancer, would choose so selfishly not to come to the aid, as we are able, of those so like us who suffer now as we have? Where those presently dealing with diagnosis and treatment experience fear of what is to come, we can impart loving reassurance, born of our own experiences; hope to dispel their doubts by reminding them, tangibly, that treatments can be effective and that most cancers are treatable; and community or fellowship where they may feel lonely in their struggle. It is incumbent upon us, as survivors, not to offer false, but authentic hope that persons currently facing their own cancer treatments, may also one day become survivors as well. With the stories we have to tell of our own experiences also comes wisdom and with the imparting of that wisdom rests hope for others. Let us not "waste" the suffering we have endured by rejecting an opportunity to give hope to others. I often refer to "hope" as "the most neglected of the theological virtues." Hope keeps us moving forward. Hearken back, if you will, to Paul's reminder to the Romans:

*"We even glory in our afflictions knowing that affliction produces endurance, and endurance, proven character, and proven character, hope, and **hope does not disappoint**…" (5:3-5).*

In the vast richness of the traditions which comprise Christian Spirituality, there is much to be said of the ever-ongoing debate regarding the synthesis of what we have come to call "the active life" and "the contemplative life." The primary biblical, and thus theological and spiritual, example of this synthesis comes from a moving section in the tenth chapter of Luke's Gospel. In this passage, you may recall that the faithful find Jesus welcomed to stay in the home of Martha as He passes through town. While there, Martha remains hard at work in the kitchen preparing the meal, likely to be served that evening. Her sister, Mary, however attentively remains at the feet of Jesus listening to the wisdom He imparts. Perturbed at a point that she has been left by her sister to bear the full burden of the chores, Martha questions Jesus, asking, *"Lord, don't you even care that my sister has left it to me to do all this work. Tell her to help me!"* Jesus then replies, *"How anxious you are about so many things. Mary has chosen the better part and it will not be taken from her" (Luke 10:38-42)*. In this example, we can observe that Martha represents the "active" spiritual life as she is, despite being anxious, still being of service to others while Mary represents the "contemplative" spiritual life by clinging to Jesus' Words of wisdom and insight. With relevance to cancer-survivorship, we can draw upon the spiritual wisdom of both Martha and Mary's examples as their respective spiritualties. True, Jesus seems to value one over the other at that particular moment, but context remains ever important. To the extent that the pursuit of "active spirituality" excludes the contemplative such that it provokes anxiety, such activity should be tempered by an embrace of the contemplative. Similarly, should one's spiritual life be entirely steeped in contemplation to the exclusion of activity and thus lead to "contemplative burn-out," "spiritual dryness," or even an aversion to meaningful labor (which need not always be manual or physical), it ought to be tempered by the embrace of the active.

Following along these parameters, we can identify and categorize some actions and activities related to embracing one's life as a cancer-survivor as part of a life of meaningful service to others, and thus, to God, whose image is reflected in each person. 1) Fundraising, 2) serving as awareness and research advocates / participants, and 3) not neglecting our continued personal health are all active means of living life as a survivor which contain within them opportunities to help others still fighting their own battles with cancer. By not neglecting to receive regular check-ups and cancer screenings as well as remaining closely attentive to our own personal health, we honor the Holy Spirit who dwells in the "Temple" of our bodies (cf. 1 Corinthians 6:19). Moreover, if we neglect our health, we needlessly risk our lives. We can be of no practical help to others in their cancer journeys if we aren't around to do so. Just as well, in the "second chances" at life we've been given, we can endeavor to make better the lives of our sisters and brothers in the cancer struggle by acting as both advocates for and participants in research. Research is crucial in the cancer world because there are a plethora of types and as such, even more a plethora of ways in which it can come to be treated. However, not all treatments are yet fully effective and until they are, our advocacy for or participation in research which could lead to greater successful outcomes is a service to those who could later be saved by the outcomes which come from our help. Through it may seem indirect makes no difference against the irrefutable fact that our help, as part of a collective whole, can make the cancer experience more positive and safer for our fellow human beings. The good that we do for them, we do also for God Himself, even if we don't always understand or see this reality. Moreover, by engaging actively in fundraising, we also assist the application of research findings into practical treatments for others who most need them.

All of these aforementioned very active means of assisting others through our own survival have three more contemplative counterparts. These three include: 1) remembering and honoring both those who have helped us along during our own confrontations with cancer (living or passed), 2) never suppressing the memories of our own cancer-journey, but instead utilizing those memories as motivation to live in the fullness of life, and 3) by facilitating or participating in cancer-related support groups. All three of these may be classified as contemplative in that before any of the fruits of these actions can ever extend outwardly to the help of others, they first require a personal investment of both mind and soul. Furthermore, what makes any act a contemplative one, at least in the Christian spiritual tradition, is that the thoughts, emotions, senses, and locutions which come from deep, interior reflection on the subjects of thought, when considered to be in dialogue with God and intentionally given over to the guidance, direction, and promptings of the Holy Spirit, can in fact, be considered a very intimate form of prayer. Indeed, from this understanding, all three of the above named actions may well be considered prayers so long as one willfully accepts God into their accompanying interior reflection.

Let us take the time now to consider not only how we may welcome God into these activities-of-thought related to our own cancer survival, but also how He has always been present in them, often their Source, even without our consciously knowing. In the first case, that is, making it a point to remember and honor those who helped us in our own confrontation with cancer as well as our sisters and brothers in the cancer struggle who have gone before us: we greet and honor the Holy Presence of God in our lives by recalling of each of these persons that most fundamental of theological and spiritual truths. As we have continuously repeated throughout this book, each of us is "created in the image and likeness of God" (Gen. 1:27). To that end, each person we encounter is an opportunity to welcome God into our lives, but still there is more. "Christ-likeness" may best be described or explained by one's demonstration or exhibition of qualities either enacted by or of value to Jesus Christ Himself. Hand-in-hand goes "Christ-likeness" with developing and practicing an ethics of imitation and devotion. What this means is this: Because Jesus loves us to so great an extent – literally, He loves us to death, "even death on a cross" (Phil. 2:8) – the only fitting response on our behalf, in return for so great a love, is love itself. In fact, St. John of the Cross well-encapsulated this onus-of-response when he wrote:

Love is repaid by love alone.

When we consider how we may, in a fitting way, simultaneously greet and welcome God's ever-abiding Presence into our contemplative reflection on those who have helped us in our own cancer journeys as well as those who have passed away from cancer, we might do well to consider the ways in which these persons "were as Christ" to us in our times of need. How were they compassionate to us as Christ is compassionate? Were they selfless in caring for us even before themselves as Christ is selfless? Did they love us when the pains of our illness and treatment made us less-than-lovable just as Christ loves us even in our darkest hours? There are countless other means by which those who cared for us or have passed on before us may have acted in Christ-like ways towards us. However, in so much as they ever did to us, we have, in a way, seen reflected in them the very face of Love Himself. Such love calls out to us to respond accordingly and as we previously noted, "Love is repaid by love alone."

Here, then, is where the ethics of imitation and devotion enter in. Christian acknowledge that both the perfect example and definition of authentic love is found in the teachings, life, death, and Resurrection of Jesus. Many of us assume that perfect exhibitions of love on this side of eternity by any human being are impossible. In that way, we are not Christ, this is true, but even the name and our identity as "Christians" gives us hope. The word, "Christian" itself, after all, means, "little Christ." Insofar as our love for Jesus compels us to <u>imitate</u> His actions of forgiveness, selflessness, prayerfulness, and love, we reflect God's image and truly act as "little Christs." Of course, there is but one God made human, and so to keep in-check our pride such that we never dare to think of ourselves equal to Christ in whom we imitate by action, we willfully <u>devote</u> ourselves to His sovereignty, guidance, protection, and continual inspiration. In sum, reflecting on those who have helped us in our own battle against cancer, in any ways they have, is a means of reflecting upon the eternal goodness of God also, whose Divine Image is so beautifully reflected in those who, often disregarding self, thought first of us in our times of greatest need.

      The second means of contemplative spiritual reflection in our survival are the opportunities to embrace, as motivating sources, our memories of our cancer experiences rather than to suppress or "run-away" from those memories. Very often, memories of negative experiences, while sometimes initially frightening or painful, have within them the capabilities to stir-up in us a desire for change. In the case of those of us who have experienced cancer, perhaps our own sometimes difficult memories can be harnessed into a renewed zest for life as well as the desire to lessen the sufferings of others still going through what we have already overcome. I personally know how painful the memories of cancer experiences can be. Full disclosure: I was recently (at the time of this writing) even diagnosed with a most mild form of PTSD, relating to my past cancer struggles and my occasional concerns of its return or the occurrence of subsequent terminal illnesses. Be that as it may, I have found some strength and comfort through the contemplative embrace of my memories. The hard truth is that as much as we may want to suppress, escape, or forget our more painful memories, we actually, in so attempting to do so, cause further emotional and sometimes even spiritual harm to ourselves. Rather than doing this, we might consider allowing our negative memories to become prayerful reflections themselves. According to Drs. Andrew Newberg and Mark Waldman in their splendid and captivating book, <u>How God Changes Your Brain</u> (2010), contemplation or "meditation undermines the everyday doubts and anxiety we all harbor when we reach for new goals and ideals" (pg. 165). If our new goals and/or ideals are, as we previously mentioned, to glorify God with a new zest for life and help lessen the sufferings of others, then perhaps over time, our painful memories of the past, lessened in anxiety through prayerful contemplation and meditation, may actually become catalysts which help us attain to these goals. Further thoughtfulness about our own cancer experiences also has the potential, as paradoxical as this may initially seem, to motivate us by reminding us of our own mortality. When we consider our previous proximity to death and look presently at our renewed life, we may feel compelled to live more vibrantly and with even more purpose or "gusto" than before. Such inspiration can be welcomed into the spiritual life as the Holy Spirit's prompting through one's situations-in-life to live as one may not have lived before. After all, it was St. Irenaeus of Lyon who said, *"The glory of God is humanity fully alive."*

The final mean of engaging contemplatively with our cancer survival is via the medium of either participation in or facilitation of a cancer-related, or cancer-survival specific, support group. This may seem, at the outset, misplaced in categorization as a contemplative spiritual practice rather than an active one, but hopefully you will come to see its contemplative roots as we proceed. Here seems like as good a place as any to mention two important pieces of information; both of which have direct relevance both to the universal cancer experience and to the practice of Christian spirituality as a whole and thus, comprising both, this entire book:

> 1) Spirituality is about and finds its genesis in "lived-experiences."

> 2) It is a subject that demands personal involvement between God, ourselves, and others.

Cancer is never the "stuff of theory." It is an unfortunate reality that, to truly understand, can only be experienced. In my own life, I feel like I sometimes come across to persons as rather condescending when I mention that a person who has never had cancer might never understand fully its multidimensional complexities. Condescending or not, there is much truth in that statement. We would not pretend to fully understand the horrible pains of a sexual-assault victim; nor should we with persons who have faced cancer – unless, of course, we have similarly experienced their trials ourselves. Should we not have personally experienced such adversities, our best efforts would be harnessed into developing empathy, compassion, and availing ourselves to learn from the person who has encountered the adversities. Though it is most often said with well-meaning intention by persons trying to be supportive of cancer-affected persons, the phrase, "I understand," can actually be perceived by the cancer-affected person as a most callous statement given that in order to truly understand the adversities faced by cancer-affected persons, one must have experienced such adversities for oneself. Unless one has done so, it is apparently clear that they do not actually or truly understand and instead what a person means to say is: "Help me understand." So, just as cancer is entirely experiential; that is, it is different for each person, so also is spirituality as a whole. Cancer-spirituality, then, is a most varied subject. This book cannot address all experienced unique to each individual, but just as one must continually return to the feet of the Savior, my hope is that, especially since this book's contents point ever to the Savior Himself, you might find reason to continue returning to it as a guide in developing your spiritual relationship with God, yourself as a cancer-survivor, and others whom you have been "called" to assist in their own spiritual journey.

Whether you come to utilize this book within a support-group context or not, I cannot overemphasize how valuable cancer-related support groups can be. In them, you will meet others who have, though somewhat differently most likely, come to have shared similarly in the unique complexities of the cancer experience. Meeting and connecting with these persons will allow you the opportunities to share insights from your own experience and to learn from theirs. This builds one another up and therefore is wholly constructive. Moreover, support groups afford the chances for participants to pray for and with one another – a most valuable gift and help in the Christian spiritual life. The importance and value of community in the spiritual life can also not be understated, and obviously, support groups do not occur in isolation, but as their name implies, within small groups that form and make-up communities. Experiencing various aspects of life with others not only affords us opportunities to obtain perspective, but to encounter others who have encountered also what we have and who do so live to us as evidence that we need not face our journeys alone. Apart from encountering Christ reaching out into our lives in the care and support of others, we may also call to mind that Jesus valued community so greatly that we might even come to think of His Twelve Apostles as perhaps "the world's first support-group." By their example, may we never forget to keep Christ at the center of our own groups as well.

Finally, if this longer-than-usual chapter leaves us with only one (but, hopefully more than one) learned-idea, it is my hope that it will be this:

Having been created by Love, out of love, our duty is to return love chiefly to God and to all His human creation, and therefore, for this reason, our lives are not our own.

Just a paragraph ago, I mentioned the Apostles of Jesus. Well, even if difficult sometimes to see or comprehend how possible, <u>we</u> (yes, each of us) are spiritual successors to the Apostles and, as such, have upon our shoulders a similar mission to which we are entrusted. Before ascending into Heaven, Jesus gathered His Apostles and to them (as well as each of us) says:

"All power in Heaven and earth has been given to me. Go, then, into every nation and gather disciples, baptizing them in the name of the Father, and of the Son, and of the Holy Spirit, and know that I am forever with you" (Matt. 28:20).

Our survivor-status, indeed as those who have overcome cancer, is a sort of "micro-commissioning" which reflects this much larger "Great Commission." We are called to comfort, to console, to cheer, to be bearers of hope to all others who have or ever will experience the personal confrontation with cancer. If, by our own suffering, we possess the knowledge, born of experience, to lessen the sufferings of others, then we are called to do so. Our work of fighting cancer is not complete when we are cured ourselves, even though the ways we fight have changed. When Jesus ascended, His mission carried on. Like the Apostles before us who bravely carried out Jesus' mission, there is still a mission before each of us. There is still work to be done in the cancer fight so let's get to it!

Chapter 13:
The "New Normal"

"Cancer can take away all of my physical abilities.
It cannot touch my mind, it cannot touch my heart,
and it cannot touch my soul."
~ Coach Jim Valvano

I come from a family who were obviously so affected by watching my own cancer struggle that they feel it necessary to remind me even to this day that I am "perfectly normal." Of course, I know for the most part that this is a coping method for their own benefit, and I certainly don't fault them for their optimism. However, I know of a somewhat different reality. I am often fearful or anxious that my cancer will return or (thanks to the chemo I did receive) that subsequent other cancers or complications will arise. I have a personal fear of dying early (as in like before 40, may God forbid it) and as a result of these trauma-born concerns, I have a few trauma and anxiety-related disorders which also contribute to my occasional bouts with depression (which is sometimes made worse by other events known as "triggers"). My reason for mentioning all of this isn't to garner sympathy from readers, but to mention the importance of understanding that there is **_so much more_** involved in one's "normal" life after cancer of which so many others are alarmingly unaware.

Holistic-Wellness is a term which refers to all four dimensions which comprise our wellness as a human person and which include our: 1) physicality, 2) emotionality, 3) intellectuality, and perhaps most importantly, 4) spirituality. Should any of these dimensional areas of our life and personality be left "off-kilter" as a result of our cancer experiences, sure, we may try and correct them, if we so choose, but we also may be unable to always correct them **fully**. In such cases (or even in the event we choose, for whatever reason not to correct them), it is incumbent upon those who love us (significant others, friends, and family) to accept and still love (in just as compassionate and attentive a way) us as they always have, if not even more so. They must come to understand what we as survivors will always know first, namely, that we now live life in light of a "new normal." To be sure, the term "normal" or "normalcy" is a complex one. Dictionaries define "normalcy" as: *"A sense of what is usual, typical, or expected."* I say that this term is complex not because of the definition itself, but rather because of the ambiguity involved in assessing what is "usual," "typical," or "expected" from one person to another.

Consider the vast number of cancers which exist, as well as the wide array of human personalities. Add to this the multidimensional facets of each human person consisting of their physicality, emotionality, intellectuality, and spirituality and from this consideration alone, one must reasonably infer that cancer affects each person differently during their confrontation with it as well as those of us who survive it. That said, our adjustments to the "new normal" of life after cancer would do well to be met with patience with self, compassion for the well-intentioned actions of those who care for us, and a continual recollection upon the Providence of God.

Firstly, we should be patient with ourselves by recognizing that and glorying in the fact that we have, whether we are yet comfortable admitting it to ourselves or not, been _ontologically changed_ by our encounter with cancer... and I would contend, regardless of how we may feel it has "limited" us, for the better. As a result of what we have suffered, we have gained an awareness of how personally and profoundly the God of All Creation beautifully and triumphantly "makes all things new," especially since we are now living in the "newness of life" on earth.

Secondly, we must be sensitive to the well-intentioned actions of those who care for us by, at times, "giving them a pass" for not fully understanding our sufferings or even difficulties in adjusting to the "new normal" of life after cancer. That said, "willful ignorance" or a refusal to meet us in our own sensitivities on their part **demands** "correction" or "reproof" as we cancer-survivors cannot (nor should we ever even feel the need to) apologize for our needs for compassion in terms of how we interact with others given these "new normal." An illustrative example may shed some greater clarity on what I mean here. There are marked differences between someone's well-intentioned, but not always helpful attempts to be sensitive to a survivor's "new normal" and one who is "willfully ignorant" or callous all together.

Example of Well-Intentioned Attempt

Perhaps a survivor, prior to cancer, enjoyed a certain activity, place, or food and in efforts to facilitate a "return to normalcy," has a family member or friend who insists on celebrating said activity with, taking their survivor friend / relative to said place, or making them their favorite food.

If the now-survivor's memories or enthusiasm of any of these things are now somehow "tainted" by – let's say negative memories of these same things experienced through their cancer struggle, then so be it. Perhaps those things are "old normal," not "new normal" for the survivor. Still, the intention of who cares for the survivor was to bring them happiness even if unsuccessful. This is only a good thing and survivors should explain, with sensitivity toward their friend or relative, why they may no longer enjoy these things, but still express gratitude for their loved-one's care and effort.

Example of Willful-Ignorance

Perhaps as a result of one's cancer-trauma, a survivor deals with a persistent fear of death or the recurrence of their original cancer or even the development of another cancer. The survivor's friend or relative "brushes off" their concerns as overreaction or dismisses the survivor's need for emotional healthcare. Perhaps said friend or family member even dares to accuse the survivor of being "weak in faith," asserting that if only their faith were stronger, their worries would diminish.

Christian theology teaches prominently the importance of forgiveness and so we should certainly forgive these "willfully ignorant" persons of their callousness, but we are under no obligations to remain subject to actions, comments, or statements which clearly are so spiritually (and emotionally) destructive. If, after an attempt has been made to correct, in charity and love, the negative impact of the actions, the wisdom of Jesus to the Apostles is most fitting should said person(s) persist in their "willful ignorance." The Lord reminds us:

"Whomever does not receive you or heed your words, depart from them then, and shake the dust from your feet" (Matt 10:14).

Having suffered, as we have, so greatly from our cancer, we need not suffer needlessly any further, especially at the hands of others. In this way, we faithfully affirm our own human dignity, value, and worth as persons created *imago Dei*. It is also a conducive step towards positive self-love and self-care.

Thirdly and most importantly, our adjustments to the "new normal" of life post-cancer can and will be more richly and fruitfully solidified through continual recollection on the Divine Providence of God. Adjusting or readjusting to anything new is never an easy task. We will encounter struggles along the way and God is fully aware of this. He is patient with us and abundant in mercy. St. Francis de Sales, easily one of the most positive and uplifting spiritual writers of the faith has even before written:

> *"When human efforts fail, all is not wanting; for God takes over and cares for us by His special providence."*

Nowhere else is God's "special" or "Divine" providence more clear than in three gifts He constantly showers upon us. These three gifts are known as "the theological virtues," and consist of 1) Faith, 2) Hope, and 3) Love. Cancer may well have changed us and forced us into learning to accept the "new normal," but hearken back if you will to the opening quote of this chapter. Coach Jim Valvano said, "Cancer… cannot touch my soul." Neither can it touch ours and even if everything else in our life after cancer seems different or even if we have "fallen away" from them for a while, it nevertheless remains true that *"faith, hope, and love remain, these three" (1 Cor. 13:13)* and they remain in us as the most powerful helpers of all – true gifts from God – to help us embrace, enjoy, and even attain happiness in living the "new normal." As we continue this chapter, providing a sort of survey-overview of the value of embracing the theological virtues as a survivor, I will frequently be quoting from and drawing upon insights from the brilliant and well-researched book entitled, _Cancer: A Medical and Spiritual Guide for Patients and their Families_ (2004) by William Fintel, M.D. and Gerald McDermott, Ph.D. I am indebted to both of these persons and highly recommend their book as supplemental reading to this one. Drs. Fintel, McDermott, and I all agree that even as survivors "have won the physical battle against cancer, their lives will be changed irrevocably" (pg. 310). That said, we must acknowledge as Christian faithful, that we are not only physical beings and as such, it is often, especially in life after cancer, not chiefly our bodies that need to continue to heal, but our emotions and our souls as well.

The first of the theological virtues – faith – is our belief in Jesus Christ, true God and true man. It is by faith that we enter into and continue in our relationship with God. This relationship is, of course, made stronger by prayer. In any phase of the cancer journey, faith assures us of both the true Presence of and abiding help from the One who can and does intervene when all human efforts, including our own, seem to come up short. Drs. Fintel and McDermott write:

"Patients with faith know that ultimately they cannot depend on human beings alone for recovery, but that God is the ultimate Source of health" (pg. 266).

It is for this reason, after all, that God is often referred to as "the Divine Physician." When struggling to adjust to the "new normal" of life post-cancer, faith beckons us to ask God for help as we continue our recovery. Sometimes it is truly as simple as merely asking. Remember to remain persistent in prayer and never neglect continuing to pray even when things seem to have improved.

In my theological and chaplaincy careers, I have often taken to referring to "hope" as the most underestimated of the theological virtues. Everyone speaks of faith and even more so of love, but poor "hope"… it often gets lost in the mix. This has always shocked me a bit, especially since St. Paul himself assures us that *"hope does not disappoint" (Romans 5:5).* Admittedly, that one may be a "tough-sell" for some, especially those who may have hoped for a loved-one's healing only for them to pass on or for ones who have hoped that a relationship be salvaged only for it to inevitably end in separation. However, in such trying circumstances when hope seems all but defeated, I often remember something St. Thomas More said. He wrote, *"Earth has no sorrow that Heaven cannot heal."* For me at least, this quote inspires seeing hope in light of the temporary versus the enduring-eternal. Consider this: When we lose loved ones (either to death or emotional separation), do we, as Christian people, sincerely believe that's all there is to it? Or, do we believe that an eternal reunion awaits us where all the sad and earthly divisions which separate us will be no more? For me at least, I know the loss of people I love pushes me to "press-on" even stronger in the hope of being forever reunited with them in Heaven. Earthly hopes, then, may disappoint, but ultimate hope… that never disappoints. One of the most difficult aspects in the "new normal" of cancer-survivorship is combatting feelings of hopelessness (either from "survivor's guilt" or the belief that one may never again know happiness as one did prior to diagnosis). Of this notion, Drs. Fintel and McDermott provide further insight, noting: *"A sense of hopelessness can be overcome by appealing to the Source of all hope – the Living God" (pg. 138).*

As the expression goes, we've "saved the best for last." Not only does St. Paul say, in reference to the final theological virtue, that *"the greatest of these is love" (1 Cor. 13:13)*, but even St. John says with even greater telling-force, *"God is Love" (1 Jn. 4:8).* Love is the very nature of God and as such, God's very Spirit is present wherever there is authentic, selfless, and unconditional love. So powerful even is love that the theologian, William of St. Thierry wrote of its power to fundamentally change and give value to what is loved. He said, *"When a soul reaches out in love to anything, a change takes place by which it is transmuted into the object loved."* If, then, we are facing difficulties embracing any aspects of the "new normal" of post-cancer life, let us attempt, with greater fervor, to love God, to love others, and to even love ourselves regardless – or better yet – in spite of what we believe our imperfections to be. *"Love, forgiveness, and the will-to-live are related to one's ability to survive cancer" (pg. 204)*, write Drs. Fintel and McDermott; to which I would add, "as well as to thrive after cancer." Before closing out this chapter, I believe it worth mentioning that the theological virtues mirror the Holy Trinity in their inseparability. Faith draws us to belief in God in whom there is the ultimate fulfillment of what is hoped for, and all of this proceeds from the inexhaustible fount of Christ's self-giving Love for each one of us personally.

Suggested Spiritual Exercises & Further Resources
Part III

1) Examine as best as your memory will allow how you lived life prior to diagnosis. Did you simply exist in body (βίος) or did you live life to its fullest (ζωή)?

   *- Write a list of at least 6 ways (2 for each category below) in which you will live in the "fullness of life" (ζωή) relating more vibrantly with **God, Others,** and **Yourself.***

2) By virtue of our cancer-survival, we have been "called" to serve a particular mission; that is, to help our fellow sisters and brothers still fighting cancer in and throughout their journeys. Because they are created in God's image as we also have been, we also honor God by being of help to them.

   *- Reflect on ways in which you can and will "give back" from your own second-chance at life for the benefit of others. Write down 1 way each that you will prayerfully or practically give of yourself from your **time, talents,** and **treasures.***

3) Try to identify one element of your life that is part of your "new normal" of life after cancer.

   *- In **Faith**, ask God in prayer to help you adjust to it more fully.*

   *- Give **Hope** to someone else by reminding them that they need not face their cancer journey alone.*

   *- Acknowledge your new "fullness of life" as an outgrowth of God's **Love** for you.*

4) Consider reading:

   - <u>Cancer Journey: A Caregiver's Guide from the Passenger Seat</u> by Cynthia Zahm Siegfried

   - <u>The Inner Voice of Love</u> by Henri Nouwen

- *Cancer: A Medical and Spiritual Guide for Patients and their Families* by *William Fintel, M.D. and Gerald McDermott, Ph.D.*

5) Listen to a Podcast episode of "Eternal Insight" entitled, *"Cancer & Spirituality"* at the permanent link listed below:

- **https://itunes.apple.com/us/podcast/eternal-insight/id1273491058?mt=2&i=1000394300716**

6) Visit and explore the website of the National Coalition for Cancer Survivorship.

- *www.canceradvocacy.org*

Chapter 14:
Take Courage!

When I began writing this concluding chapter for this book, it marked exactly one year since the sudden and ultimately unexpected passing of one of my best friends. The evening before the one-year anniversary of his going to Heaven, I attended Sunday Mass for the Feast of Christ the King of the Universe. Listening to the priest's homily, my mind could not help but think back on the past memories of times spent with my friend. Usually, I am a very attentive listener to lectures, homilies, sermons, whatever you choose to call them, but this time, as I've discovered, my memories were nurtured by the Holy Spirit who imparted wisdom of which no homily alone would have been capable. Noticing the priest's movements during the homily, I was "snapped out" on occasion of the deep reminiscence about my friend and was still able to absorb "bits and pieces" of the wisdom he was imparting. On this Feast of Christ the King, he was explaining the moving story and heroic virtue of a soon-to-be Mexican saint, Miguel Agustin Pro.

Pro was a Jesuit priest who, during the persecution of Christians in Mexico in 1927, was executed by authority of the Mexican President at that time for refusing to recant of his faith. Standing before a firing squad, just before they shot, Pro, already holding a cross in his right hand, raised both of his arms in cruciform fashion and loudly shouted, "Viva Cristo Rey!" With his courageous exclamation (which translated from Spanish means, "Long Live Christ the King!"), Pro was executed, but died a martyr and a living witness to the sovereignty of the incarnate-God and Ruler of All. The final words of the priest's homily reminded me of my own friend and were deeply profound. He said, *"No one will willingly die for something they know to be a lie, but they will for Truth. Even if they know it's true, still, that takes courage!"* My friend, though his life was short, lived courageously. He lived in a way which assured that, like him or not, you would not forget him. He made me want to live more courageously myself and so, not only is this book partially dedicated to him, but this chapter is, I believe in a real way, inspired by his memory. That said, I proceed.

Courage, indeed, sisters and brothers! Courage, indeed. Even the Lord Himself told us: *"In this world, you will have trouble, but take courage, I have overcome this world"* *(Jn. 16:33).* I often read and meditated upon these Words and thought to myself, "Well good for Jesus that He overcome the world, but I'm not Him so why should I have courage that I can overcome what troubles me?" Obviously, my faith is not perfect and never will be on this side of eternity, but my answer to that nagging question continues to become clearer each time I pray. It is *precisely* because I am **not** Jesus that I can, should, and do have any hope at all of overcoming the trials of this life. I never could overcome them on my own, but I am made in the image of the One who can and who does. By faith in, hope for, and love of Jesus, and in the words of Blessed Oscar Romero of El Salvador,

"We as Christians will not fail for we bear the Spirit that raised Jesus to new life" (1978).

That said, if this Person in whom we believe has truly overcome even death, and we have that same Spirit within us, then already *"we are more than conquerors through Him who loved us" (Romans 8:37).*

When I lost my friend in his death and a few months later, another person very dear to me (this time in emotional separation), courage to press-on was quite difficult for me to find. Truth be told, I still struggle somewhat with both of these today. However, Jesus' Words come with something much more than merely "cheery optimism" or a "self-help-mantra." His Words contain within them not only Divine Providence, but also unfailing promise. That very promise, sometimes implicit, but also over overt, in Jesus' Words and teachings evokes courage and is especially relevant to all persons who have ever or will ever encounter cancer. For this reason, namely, that courage is a unifying force for those who have lost loved-ones to cancer, those currently fighting their own battle with it, and for survivors, this chapter rests outside of parts I, II, or III of this book. It can and quite literally, as the courage it takes to bear witness to Truth often does, stands on its own. Before we explore the ways in which courage is so central to our overcoming any confrontations related to cancer, we first must authentically understand the importance of promises – from out of which our courage emanates.

As a segue into this discussion, I remember once before seeing an unattributed quote which was shared by a friend of mine on the popular social media platform, Twitter. The quote, short but poignant, read: "People ask me why it's so hard to trust others, and I ask them, why is it so hard to keep a promise?" What this quote reveals (given the fact that it had been shared over two-hundred forty thousand times) more than anything are that deep wounds, heartbreak, depression, anxiety, and yes, even fear (the vice against courage) all stem from both personal and collective negligence in truly coming to honor promises and commitments. Our world and culture has been successful in deceiving so many of us into the belief that promises, commitments, or even vows are valid or to be honored only so long as we *feel* like doing so. The moment, however, a promise or the like causes us any discomfort, inconvenience, perceived restriction of freedom, or exacts a price from us, we have sadly and oh so inaccurately come to believe that on these grounds we have rights to terminate or "break" our promises without any guilt or regret. But, what of the human persons (bearers always of God's image and likeness as we are) who are impacted by these broken promises, commitments, or vows? According to Professor Stephen Carter in his book on and thus entitled, <u>Integrity</u>, "Saint Augustine contended that any promise not kept was a sin against God's gift of speech" (pg. 33). No wonder there is such fear, anguish, heartbreak, sadness, and distrust in our world today.

Cancer patients learn especially quickly that promises of cures or good health are rarely made. This is because their caregivers understand the drastic emotional toll that broken promises can have on the persons to whom the promises fail to come to fruition. Instead of promises of cures, patients receive promises of supportive presence, of prayer, and of continual perseverance despite the adversity that comes along. One would think that is persons can promise such beautiful emotional and spiritual support in times of catastrophic illness that it would be even easier to promise (and actually fulfill) what was promised in happier circumstances. St. Camillus de Lellis, founder of the religious order in Italy which cared for the sick and was actually the original Red Cross before it was secularized once said this of promises and commitments:

> *"Commitment is doing what you said you'll do after the feelings you said it in have passed."*

De Lellis seized on a necessary and oft-neglected facet of promise-keeping, and even authentic love itself. Keeping one's promises and loving persons both are entirely matters of constant and continual choice and have little to nothing to do with feelings. A hard reality-check for many, to be sure; for in this day and age, the vast majority improperly view love, promises, and commitments all through the fleeting lenses of "feelings" or emotions. But, while feelings and emotions are subject-to-change, promises, commitments, and love bear, at all times regardless of human awareness or intent, the foundational changelessness and constancy of their Divine Author and example par excellence about whom sacred scripture notes: *"Jesus Christ is the same yesterday, today, and forever"* *(Hebrews 13:8).*

What, then, does all this talk of promises have to do with courage and overcoming experiences with cancer? Let me offer this: In the world of cancer diagnosis, treatment, grief, or survival, very seldom are promises made and even less are they kept. We become so used to disappointments or "let-downs" during our cancer experience. But, in life after cancer, if we ever hope to overcome or dispel the darkness of disappointment, hopelessness, or isolation, we must dare to be courageous! And what is more courageous than living boldly and unashamedly for Christ's Kingdom in a world and culture that has tried and continues to try so hard to overthrow the One who rules over all in the first place? The Kingdom of God is not only that into which we hope to enter when we go to Heaven, but it also stretches to the here and now. Christ is King of both Heaven **_and_** earth. We all are His citizens and are charged with ushering in the eternal reign of Christ, the King, here on earth and in our own lives. Promises – making them and keeping them – to God and to one another is only but part of life within His Kingdom. Theologian Lewis Smedes, in a beautiful sermon entitled, *The Power of Promises*, said:

> *"We are never more like God than when we forgive and when we keep a promise."*

Forgiveness and faithfulness (that which is merely another way of saying "promise-keeping") are both acts of love and love, apart from being God's very nature, is also the governing law of Christ's eternal Kingdom.

Whether grief over lost loved-ones, our own personal confrontation with cancer, or painful memories we still harbor as survivors, it is courageous living that will help us overcome. This courageousness means something different for each group discussed throughout this book and largely, the work of discovering how you personally will live courageously for Christ and others will be your own. However, I hope the contents I have presented in this book have at least provided some spiritual direction. For good measure, I would like to provide, here below, a brief series of suggestions for each group discussed in the three parts that comprise this work, in terms of what we have more specifically discussed in this chapter. Drawing on Smedes quote, it is imperative that we never think of ourselves as equal to God, but that we likewise understand that imitating the sorts of qualities

God values is spiritually beneficial and draws us closer to Him in relationship in the process. That said, each group of persons discussed in this book as "touched" by cancer has an opportunity to begin to or more so live courageously by forgiving, keeping promises, and loving. Here is but one suggestion for each group as to how to practically live this spirituality:

For Those Who Have Lost Loved-Ones to Cancer:

Forgive yourself of any guilt in terms of thinking of how you could have been a better loved-one to the person you've lost. They have long since forgiven you. Instead of guilt, promise them your prayers and continued spiritual unity.

For Those Currently Battling Cancer:

Cancer is never anyone's fault. Not yours, not your loved-one's, and not God's, but we can still feel anger at cancer itself. Forgive your cancer. Yes, it sounds silly and odd, but forgive it. The angrier you remain at your cancer, the more power you give it to rob you of your joy. Instead of anger towards your cancer (or even the fact that you have it), promise to care for yourself as best you can by finding at least one reason daily for which to thank God.

For Cancer-Survivors:

We know how fragile life is. Spend no more time of your "new life" fearing disappointment. Forgive whomever has hurt you in the past and promise to never give up on loving people now. Disappointments don't stop after cancer, but you were stronger than cancer so you also are stronger than disappointment. Love boldly.

My greatest hope is that one day there will be almost no need for this book as cancer will have been ultimately defeated through eradication. Until that day dawns, however, know that all of us – all persons "touched" by cancer in whatever ways we have been – are united in both the bonds of unique experience and in the "joyful hope" of the greatest of all promises. Long before His own suffering, death, or Resurrection, Jesus made all of us a promise Himself:

"For this is the will of my Father... that everyone who believes in me may have eternal life, and I will raise them up on the last day" (Jn. 6:40).

If Jesus would have died and never risen Himself, we would have no reason to hope in this promise for each one of us. But, of course, there is good news for all of us, isn't there? Jesus' own Resurrection was proof of His ability to and intent to keep all the promises He has made to us. He is, at once, both eternal promise-maker and eternal promise-keeper. Since He has promised us life, let us live in its certainty. Let us live it abundantly!

Appendices

I.
Article:
"Of Soldiers, Survival, & Strength Unfailing"

II.
Article:
"The Soul of Survival"

III.
Prayers Inspired by the Illustrations

Appendix 1:
Of Soldiers, Survival, & Strength Unfailing

What follows is a reprint, with permission, of an article previously published by Anthony Maranise in <u>The Galleon</u>, a journal of editorial commentary and popular culture housed at Christian Brothers University in Memphis, TN.

Original date of publication: 22 September, 2016

Earlier this month, I had the pleasure of attending the Annual *Survivor's Day* event at St. Jude Children's Research Hospital in Memphis, TN. After a keynote presentation and welcome, offered by St. Jude's medical director, Dr. James Downing, the faculty of St. Jude's After Completion of Therapy (ACT) clinic along with the director of cancer survivorship, commenced the annual survivorship pinning ceremony.

The program began with a reading of the most recent "class of survivors" (those from 2000 – present day), and a number of children and teens were called by name. Once they arrived at the stage, various doctors we all knew and grew to love and respect over the years, greeted us with smiling faces and warm embraces as they affixed the survivor milestone lapel pins to each of our collars.

After some time had passed, my decade was finally called. I am a "survivor from the 90's," but this year was truly special for me. It marks 20 years of having been in remission from acute lymphoblastic leukemia (ALL).

For what it's worth, I should explain that the tradition of "survivor pinning" is not like anniversaries in the traditional sense. In marriage or career anniversaries, it's a common practice to ascribe a precious medal, stone, or color to the years accumulated since that particular wedding ceremony, start date, etc. For example, a "silver anniversary" is generally celebrated at 25 years, a "golden" at 50, and a "diamond" at 60.

In the world of cancer survivorship, this tradition doesn't exist—and for good reason. Even though it may seem that a couple remaining married for 25 years or a person persisting in the same career for a similar amount of time are spectacular feats in and of themselves, statistically, it is much rarer for those previously "touched" by cancer to be "long-term survivors." That said, 10 years of survival (in full remission) is considered a "silver" anniversary and 20 years, "golden" and so on, culminating in "Jubilee" at 50 years.

Given the special nature of such an occasion (and a true reason to lavishly celebrate), I couldn't help but reflect on my "Golden" anniversary of survivorship. While reminiscing about some of my more uplifting St. Jude experiences and on this whole concept of "survival" as a whole to a person whose positive-presence in my life once was, still is, and likely always will be very dear to me (currently serving as a U.S. Army ROTC cadet and to whom I happily dedicate this piece), I began to recall words and phrases common to both of us "survivors." Phrases like "fighting cancer," "fighting a battle," "winning or losing the battle against cancer," "winning or losing a war," even "casualties," revealed some distinct commonalities between all those "touched" by cancer (not just the survivors) and the soldiers who so bravely and selflessly protect, defend, and yes, even lay down their lives for others. What follows, here, are just those sorts of reflections.

There seems to be a prevailing attitude in the United States (particularly among political conservatives) that individuals who haven't experienced the horrors and atrocities of war or a combat situation could ever truly understand what it means to see, to feel, and to experience true evil. However, I would argue that to be a rather narrow-minded and superficial position at best. I have no doubt that human beings experience both moral and natural evils which cause unfathomable sufferings, and which can be just as horrific as the trials of war… and I definitely don't limit those who can, have, or will experience such evils to only those of us "touched" by cancer. However, for the purpose of these reflections, I will focus on those persons.

One of the greatest challenges in military service is the ethos of "service over self" in often the most thankless of situations. I've often witnessed those who whisper unkind things to their surrounding persons or classify, almost automatically, that a military person must be a 'bigot' or 'war-monger,' simply because of their preconceived (and often inaccurate) ideologies about soldiers or military personnel. The reality is that soldiers serve, willingly, to protect the rights enjoyed by those who speak against them. That is authentic selflessness. But, what of those "touched" by cancer?

I once read an op-ed in a Memphis-area publication that rather snidely revealed the contributing writer's perceived notions of the community's long-standing interest in both Le Bonheur and St. Jude. This individual wrote: "Being a cancer patient doesn't make you any more special than any other child." First of all, believe it or not, I wholeheartedly agreed with the writer's statement, but then again, I don't know a lot of persons "touched" by cancer who think of themselves as being as special as this writer insinuated. Many of us wish we would never have had to face what we have. But, we are stronger because of it. In this way, I see soldiers and survivors viewed as a very undervalued and "taken for granted" population. I've often heard it said that "A soldier prays for peace, but trains for war;" likewise, the survivor prays in thanksgiving for good health, but remains ever fearful that "the enemy" will return once again, and takes steps to live a healthy lifestyle in preparation for that return.

Secondly, both military service persons and cancer patients must endure a struggle. Though different, neither sort of struggle is one-dimensional. Military personnel as well as cancer patients must "fight" through physical, emotional, intellectual, and spiritual "battles" if they wish to "emerge victorious." The endurance of these "battles" requires both the cultivation of a substantial interior and exterior strength of body and spirit, and a strength that pre-dates their enlistment or diagnosis.

The other side of the struggles that both cancer survivors and soldiers face is the demands of self-sacrifice. The soldier who so dearly loves his/her significant other must face an "emotional onslaught" by remaining distanced from them for periods of time—either in training or in deployment. Likewise, for the cancer patient community (particularly at a research-based institution like St. Jude) patients are asked to participate in clinical trials that have the potential to lead to discoveries that could heal future cancer patients. Imagine a world where each soldier chose to "look-out" for only themselves or each cancer patient chose to "care for" themselves by resisting participation in clinical trials or research studies that could be helpful to medical professionals in their approach to treating cancer in the future. I know from lived experience that patients do have freedoms to choose certain courses of action in their care—whether that be a willingness to participate in the "full spectrum" of treatment possibilities, or to holistically care for themselves by offering details of their cancer experience to researchers. By inviting medical professionals into their cancer journey to advance the possibility of either their own treatment, the patient creates an opportunity for others to get better.

The "casualties" of both war and illness would be so much greater where it not for such selfless sacrifice and willingness to face, endure, and overcome the multi-dimensional struggles associated with each.

The U.S. Coast Guard and the Boy Scouts of America have a similar motto: "always ready/prepared." In terms of preparedness, I am relatively certain that there is no amount of training that adequately prepares any soldier or military service member for the horrors of warfare and human conflict. However, at least they are provided with training and some semblance of "what to expect" in their service. For those whose lives have been, are currently, or ever will be "touched" by cancer, there is no preparation. There is no training. There is no guarantee.

It is perhaps that final statement, "there is no guarantee," that most profoundly unites both soldiers and survivors. Both groups of persons enter into their respective "battles" with a deep sense of uncertainty and are buoyed only by hope. Cancer patients hope to either attain healing and a better "quality of life" or to be finally "released" from their sufferings. Similarly, soldiers hope to remain safe in combat situations and return home in one piece to the lives they have left "on hold" while serving abroad. In my estimation and personal experience, there is nothing that requires greater strength than entering into the "absolute unknown," but doing so with hope which might even, for the sake of another, demand of you all that you have.

I feel it's important to mention that in the world of cancer survivorship, anyone who has been "touched" by cancer (whether they're currently fighting, attained remission, or even those left to carry on without their loved one) is considered "a survivor." We're united by those experiences, and join a global community for the rest of our lives. Military personnel also form this sort of "fraternal bond" through their combat experiences. I feel fortunate to have been given the opportunity to witness both bonds—one from personally having lived it and the other from the confidence of another who is living it—I would argue that in the bravery with which they fight, every survivor is a soldier. Likewise, through the selfless sacrifices with which they also fight, every soldier is a survivor. For both, we ought to offer our most profound gratitude and admiration.

The author dedicates this piece to Mirjana Michelle Walther of Bellevue, Nebraska, currently attending Creighton University, in pursuit of both her U.S. Army commissioning as well as a degree in Education. Without her inspiration and mutual admiration, this piece would have remain undeveloped.

Appendix 2:
The Soul of Survival:

What follows is a reprint, with permission, of an article previously published by Emily Hines in The Galleon, a journal of editorial commentary and popular culture housed at Christian Brothers University in Memphis, TN.

Original date of publication: 21 April, 2017

Blessed is the first word that comes to mind when thinking of my cancer diagnosis. Although a cancer diagnosis is potentially devastating, I refused to look at mine that way. Within forty-eight hours of being diagnosed with Acute Promyelocytic Leukemia, I was flown to St. Jude Children's Research Hospital. When the paramedics rolled me into the hospital, tears began to stream down my face. Observing my concern, they advised me to not cry because everything was going to be okay. I looked up to them as a half-hearted smile spread across my face. As certain as I could be, I told them, "I know, I am at St. Jude and that means I am going to be okay."

From that moment forward, I began to experience complete healing through every person I met at the hospital. One person in particular was healing in a way none of my medical team could be. This man offered the reassuring gift of spiritual health. He brought the Eucharist – the Body of Christ – to me when I was lying on what could have potentially been my death bed. That man was Anthony Maranise.

Throughout my treatment at St. Jude Children's Research Hospital, I had the honor of representing the hospital as an ambassador. At one speaking engagement at a fundraising weekend in California, there was an open seating dinner. There, I met two couples from Memphis. One of the gentlemen mentioned that his son was also a survivor of leukemia. As the conversation progressed, I was informed that my fellow survivor had been, for a time, a chaplain at the hospital. Out of pure shock and curiosity, I asked what his son's name was and to see a picture of him. As God had it written, his son turned out to be Anthony Maranise, the very same person who literally brought me Jesus when I needed Him most.

After a full year since my diagnosis, I was reconnected with the man who played an instrumental role in my spiritual and thus, also, my physical healing. Immediately borrowing his father's phone, I called Anthony on FaceTime. Everyone seated at the dinner table could not believe what was providentially transpiring right before their eyes. Anthony and I recognized one another's faces immediately, and though we spoke briefly at first, neither one of us could contain our tears of joy… and apparently, nor could anyone else at the table.

Several weeks after our reconnection I received a direct message on Twitter from Anthony himself. One afternoon, at The Majestic Grille in downtown Memphis, we sat for lunch to discuss our providential meeting. In agreement that there are no such things as a coincidences, we wished to share part of our conversation with others, in the hopes that this story of faith and friendship will impart hope to others who may be struggling with the natural evils of cancer, in any form.

Anthony Maranise: What role did faith play in your struggle?

Emily Hines: I grew up in a Catholic family. My mom was director of the choir at our church growing up. Because of that, I have always been surrounded by spiritual music and so were my sisters. Music in general has always been healing to my family. When in the ambulance on my way to St. Jude, for the first time, I sang along to Oceans by Hillsong United. Listening to the lyrics, "Spirit lead me where my trust is without borders," I realized I have to have complete faith in God. Nothing I could do in that moment would stop me from experiencing cancer and cancer treatment. From that day forward I have had to give up control of my life. Many cancer patients can empathize with that loss of control. I believe many of us try to have authority over different aspects of our lives; however, the reality is only God has that complete power. With a prognosis of only living five to ten days after diagnosis, I needed to believe that God would bless me no matter my outcome. So, I did. Never question Him or His timing. Faith did not just play a role in my struggle. Faith was the center of my struggle.

AM: What is one of your happiest moments at St. Jude and what made it so?

EH: Well… every time I go back to the hospital I experience another happy moment! (That is weird to say about a hospital, I know.) Cliché as it may seem, the honest truth is that my happiest day at the hospital was September 7th, 2016 – the day I was declared cancer free! In five months to the day of diagnosis, my doctors and God rid my body of leukemia. It was a day full of happy tears and prayers of thanksgiving.

AM: Transitioning from patient to survivor, what has been most difficult for you?

EH: Finding my 'new normal' has been a significant struggle that I have yet to overcome. I have accepted that life will never be the same and I am okay with that. However, finding that 'new normal' is not as easy as I thought it would be. Nobody understands how it feels to be a cancer survivor unless you are one yourself. Finding my network of fellow young adult survivors has been my goal. I hope that once I have people to talk to who can empathize with me, then I will find a 'new normal' in their supportiveness.

In closing, to anyone affected by cancer, I offer this advice, having been through it myself: allow yourself to have 'bad days.' That's okay. However, you must, then, remember to give yourself wonderful days as well. I would always remind myself that there were sunnier days ahead and when those sunnier days did, indeed, arrive, they were all I had hoped for them to be. So long as the sun in your life continues to outshine the dreariness, know that there is hope, healing, and promise. These qualities, nurtured by faith, can and do provide strength to 'press on.' Never give up; God won't bring you this far to leave you.

Emily Hines is a survivor of Acute Promyleocytic Leukemia, treated and cured at St. Jude Children's Research Hospital from April to December of 2016. She is currently working towards earning her degree in political science from Millsaps College in Jackson, Mississippi after which she intends to continue advocating for funding for childhood cancer research.

Appendix 3:
Prayers Inspired by the Illustrations

To say that I am profoundly grateful to the illustrator of this book (for a number of reasons) would be an understatement.

She is, among her many talents, a phenomenally gifted artist.

When the illustrator sent me the finished cover and three-part interior illustrations for this book, I was at once filled with gratitude for not only her skills, but her entirely.

"Real art" touches the soul.

Her illustrations touched mine so much so that it moved me to "see" in each of her pieces, prayers.

What follows are those prayers for each group of persons "touched" by cancer and for whom each illustration corresponds to their particular portion of this book.

Images by & courtesy of "Missy" Walther
Prayer Text by Anthony Maranise

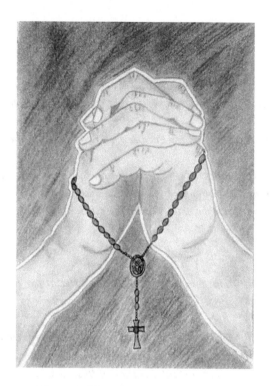

<u>*A Prayer for Those Who Have Lost Loved Ones*</u>

Sorrowful Jesus,
You who knew true sadness by Your own agony in Gethsemane's garden,
console us as we lament the loss of our loved-ones. You who knew sincere grief
at the death of Your dear friend, Lazarus, comfort us by the promise of your
Resurrection which offers us our own as well as our loved-ones'. Willfully, you
descended from the Heavenly Throne to earth to become one like us in all
things but sin. In doing so, You also chose to become broken on the cross that
You may Yourself feel and know the worst of our human brokenness. Without
You, Jesus, we are irreparable. Out of Your love, mercifully and tenderly heal
our wounds and our brokenness by reassuring us of the constancy of your
Presence and the permanence of our love for those we have lost. By Your Divine
Assistance, may we ever be linked spiritually with those we have so loved until
in the dawning of Eternal Easter, we at last, are reunited. Amen.

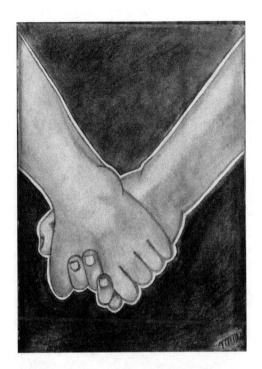

<u>A Prayer for Those Battling Cancer</u>

Jesus,
Be my strength!
So great is this adversary against me; I cannot defeat it without Your
protecting help. Only You, my God, can know the depths of my
suffering. My heart cries out to You even when I cannot find the
strength, the words, or the will to pray. But, as I do now, make me feel
Your Presence. Along Your own way of suffering, You still thought of
others as You stopped to console the weeping women of Jerusalem.
Console me now in my own afflictions that, like You, I somehow may
come to be a source of Your consolation to others. Pacify my worries,
soothe my pain, I pray. Above all, walk this road with me, Jesus, and
all for Your love's sake.
Amen.

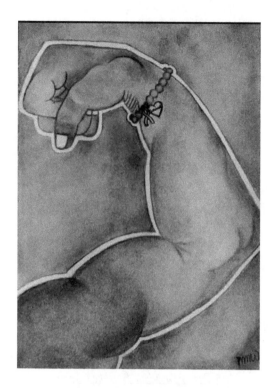

<u>*A Cancer-Survivor's Prayer*</u>

Blessed are You, Jesus Christ, the King!
In Your kindness, You have restored my physical health by the
outpouring of Your own grace and the assistance of those You have
called into Your service as healers. While you have once again made me
whole in health of body, do not cease, O Lord, to continue to strengthen
the health of my soul! Only in this health might I experience the
"fullness of life" which You have Yourself made available to all who
believe in You! Send me forth, as Your disciple, and entrusting to me a
share in Your mission of love, grant that I may use my renewed health
to help Your other children still suffering.
Amen.

Acknowledgements

Chiefly, I thank Jesus Christ Himself for granting me "newness of life." My love for and devotion to You, while at times tried by my own life's circumstances, is also that which ever pushes me forward. While I know I have (and likely will again) let you down many times, I pray that you forgive me all the more and continue to welcome me back. You are *truly* everything to me.

Of course, I gratefully acknowledge the persons to whom this book is dedicated (their primary acknowledgement is in the dedication itself), but also their families who have been so welcoming and kind to me (both the entirety of the Kraker and Walther families; for the Krakers' – Wes, Becky, Elaine, Hannah, Marie, and Wesley; and for the Walthers' – Randy, Andrea, Jeremy, Tommy, & Joey).

To Dr. Melissa Hudson, M.D., the author of this book's foreword, I thank you greatly for not only medically caring for me in my own survivorship, but for all you have cared for and continue to care for; as well as for taking time from your extremely busy schedule to write such a beautiful foreword.

To my editor who has requested anonymity, thank you as well. I know my OCD / Type-A personality made dealing with me in matters of clarity and specificity its own "cross" to bear. Nevertheless, I thank you for undertaking the task as well as for lending me your services at no cost.

In gratitude to my graphic designer, Breanna Parker: You truly have found your calling in this world. I am so impressed not only by your talents, but also by your faith and devotion to the Lord. Without you, this book would not be.

My parents, Tony & Judy, are owed a great deal of thanks as well for their continued supportiveness to me in the trying times that led to the writing of this book. They are among the first persons in whom I saw the face of Jesus Christ Himself so beautifully reflected in the way they cared for me in my own cancer journey. I love you both more than any words will ever convey and I thank you for continuing to be supportive of my works and endeavors.

To all those who provided endorsements for this book (see a complete list in the front): I cannot tell you how grateful I am to each of you for not only reading this work, but for lending your credibility, your faith, and your time to me in the hopes that your words will inspire others to give this book a chance.

*To my "inner-circle" of closest friends, David, Malorie, Kevin, and Adam: When others have walked out of my life during its most difficult times, each of you has steadfastly remained. You don't know (and may never fully) how grateful I am for each one of you guys' continuing presence in my life. God gives us friends that we do not have to carry the "crosses" of this life alone. Thank you all for helping me carry mine; and for letting me help carry yours. It's my honor.

In a special way, I acknowledge all the professors who instructed within as well as fellow graduates of the 2017 M.A. in Catholic Studies Program at CBU in Memphis. A number of my ideas contained in this book came to me as a result of our mutually shared interests in and conversations surrounding a number of theological topics.

To all persons "touched" in any way by cancer, especially children and their families of St. Jude

Children's Research Hospital in Memphis: You are not alone. God walks always with each of us, even when we doubt or fail to see how. We are all in this together and are one family united in experience. Keep fighting!

Finally, I would be remiss if I didn't thank, by name, a host of others who, in one way or another, contributed to the insights which helped make-up this book, or who acted as genuine support systems to me along the way. These persons include: My grandmothers, Gloria & Linda; grandfathers (in Heaven), Albert & Mario; Godparents, Joe & Donna; Emily Heckman; Abe Abuelouf; Suzanne Fogarty; Karissa Jacobsen; Jimmy Lucchesi; the physicians who treated me during my own battle with cancer and continue to watch over me today: Drs. Gaston Rivera, Torrey Sandlund, & Tim Folse, M.D.; The Carney Family; Fr. Jolly Sebastian; the monks and priests of St. Bernard Abbey in Cullman, AL., and my step-relatives and their families.

To anyone I may have inadvertently omitted: Please accept my apologies and "count it to my head, not to my heart." For you as well, I am grateful.

I ask that my dearest friends ensure (though I am not expecting it anytime soon, whenever that day may come) that a copy of this book is interred with me into a place of final rest as well as in addition to the other tasks I have privately asked of each of you.

Bibliography & Cited Works

Aelred of Rievaulx. *Spiritual Friendship (Text & Commentary)*. Edited by Lawrence C. Braceland and Marsha L. Dutton, Cistercian Publications, 2010.

Benedict of Nursia. *The Rule of St. Benedict*. Edited by Timothy Fry, OSB, Liturgical Press, 1981.

The New American Bible. Complete Study Ed., Fireside Publishers, 2001.

Bonhoeffer, Dietrich. *Meditations on the Cross*. Edited by Manfred Weber. Translated by Douglas W. Stott, Westminster John Knox Press, 1998.

"Cancer and Spirituality." Interview by Malorie Taff. Audio blog post. *Apple Podcasts*. Anchor FM, 1 Nov. 2017. Web. https://itunes.apple.com/us/podcast/eternalin sight/id1273491058?mt=2&i=1000394300716.

Carter, Stephen L. *Integrity*. HarperPerennial, 1997.

Catechism of the Catholic Church. Claretian Publications, 2000.

Cunningham, Lawrence, and Keith J. Egan. *Christian spirituality: themes from the tradition*. Paulist Press, 1996.

Francis de Sales. *Introduction to the Devout Life*. Vintage Books, 2002.

Fintel, William A., and Gerald R. McDermott. *Cancer: A Medical and Spiritual Guide for Patients and Their Families*. Baker Books, 2004.

Frankl, Viktor E. *Man's Search for Meaning*. Beacon Press, 2006.

Granger, Kate. "Having cancer is not a fight or a battle." *The Guardian*, Guardian News and Media, 25 Apr. 2014, www.theguardian.com/society/2014/apr/25/having-cancer-not-fight-or-battle.

Hines, Emily. "The Soul of Survival: How I Confronted Cancer with Faith." *Galleon: Digital News Magazine*, Christian Brothers University, 21 Apr. 2017, www.galleon.buzz/feed/posts/the-soul-of-survival-how-i-confronted-cancer-with-faith.

John Paul II. *On the Christian meaning of human suffering; Salvifici doloris*. Pauline Books & Media, 1984.

Lewis, C. S. *A Grief Observed*. HarperSanFrancisco, 1996.

-------------- *The Four Loves*. HarperSanFrancisco, 1981.

Maranise, Anthony. "Dr. Scott Geis on Teaching, Suffering, and Listening." *YouTube*, The Galleon, 15 Feb. 2017, www.youtube.com/watch?v=Caz3KKCzjWw.

-------------- "I've Seen the Face of God: How faith helped me survive childhood leukemia." *Magazine*, The Word Among Us, 14 June 2010,

http://wau.org/archives/article/ive_seen_the_f
ace_of_god/.

-------------- "Of Soldiers, Survivors, & Strength
       Unfailing." *Galleon: Digital News Magazine*,
       Christian Brothers University, 22 Sept. 2016,
       www.galleon.buzz/feed/posts/of-soldiers-
       survivors--strength-unfailing.

Newberg, Andrew B., and Mark Robert. Waldman. *How
       God changes your brain: breakthrough findings
       from a leading neuroscientist.* Ballantine Books,
       2010.

Nouwen, Henri J. M. *The Inner Voice of Love.* Doubleday
       Religious Pub. Group, 1999.

Siegfried, Cynthia. *Cancer Journey: A Caregiver's View from
       the Passenger Seat.* CZS Books, 2010.

Simão, Talita, et al. "The Effect of Prayer on Patients'
       Health: Systematic Literature Review."
       Religions, vol. 7, no. 1, ser. 11, 21 Jan. 2016.

Simon, Stacy. "Study: Cancer Patients with Strong
       Religious or Spiritual Beliefs Report Better
       Health." *News*, American Cancer Society, 21
       Oct. 2015, www.cancer.org/latest-news/study-
       cancer-patients-with-strong-religious-or-
       spiritual-beliefs-report-better-health.html.

Smedes, Lewis B. "The Power of Promises."
       ChristianityToday.com, Christianity Today, 1 Dec.
       2002,

www.christianitytoday.com/ct/2002/december
web-only/12-16-56.0.html.

Strobel, Lee. *The Case for Easter: A journalist investigates the Evidence for the resurrection.* Zondervan, 2014.

Watson, Nick J., and Andrew Parker. *Sports, Religion and Disability.* Routledge, 2015.

About the Author

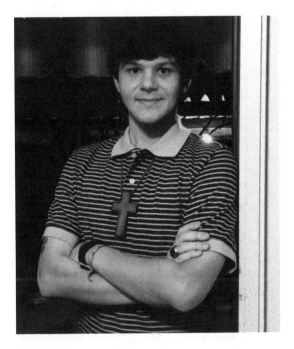

Anthony Maranise is an instructor of Religious Studies at The University of Memphis, a certified life-coach, chaplain, and is the author of 4 other books and numerous academic pieces. Primarily a theological scholar with expertise in the intersections between sports and spirituality, Anthony received his Masters from Christian Brothers University in Memphis, TN. At the time of this book's publication, he is also a 20+ year cancer survivor, treated at St. Jude Children's Research Hospital, and remains active in advocacy for advancing cancer research as well as in facilitating spiritual direction for persons affected by cancer.

To learn more about Anthony's work, visit:
http://amaranis.wixsite.com/amjm

"In our darkest hour, we are only called to love yet more gloriously."

~ Emily R. Heckman

Personal Notes:

CPSIA information can be obtained
at www.ICGtesting.com
Printed in the USA
LVHW02*1007030418
572051LV00001BA/1/P